# Irresistible Detox Elixirs

## A Love Affair with Healthful Drinks

**About the author**

**Dr. Rajat Trehan** is a passionate advocate for holistic health and well-being, empowering individuals to achieve optimal vitality through the transformative power of natural healing. Combining his extensive educational background, including a PhD in Clinical Nutrition and a Master's in Nutritional Science, with over 11 years of experience, Dr. Trehan guides his clients on a journey towards optimal health.

Fueled by a mission to spread love, joy, and happiness through the power of plants, Dr. Trehan champions a unique approach focused on addressing the root causes of lifestyle diseases. He firmly believes in leveraging the synergy of dietary changes, natural therapies, and mindful lifestyle modifications to achieve holistic and sustainable results.

Beyond his clinical practice, Dr. Trehan is a dedicated thought leader, actively educating and empowering communities across the globe. He has touched the lives of thousands by successfully reversing chronic conditions like diabetes, arthritis, and liver disorders, offering a beacon of hope for those seeking natural solutions.

Dr. Trehan's infectious enthusiasm, combined with his deep scientific knowledge and compassionate approach, make him a trusted guide on your path to vibrant health. Through his engaging lectures, workshops, and publications, including this very book, "Irresistible Detox Elixirs," he continues to inspire and empower individuals to embrace the transformative power of plant-based wellness.

# Irresistible Detox Elixirs

## A Love Affair with Healthful Drinks

Dr. Rajat Trehan

New Delhi

*Published by*
**Dr. Rajat Trehan**
B-1/626, Janak Puri,
New Delhi-110058
India
*Phone:* +91-11-47506464; 9810361459
*Email:* contact@drrajattrehan.com
*Web:* www.drrajattrehan.com

**2024**
Printed in India


**Cataloging in Publication Data--DK**
Courtesy: D.K. Agencies (P) Ltd. <docinfo@dkagencies.com>

**Trehan, Rajat, author.**
**Irresistible detox elixirs: a love affair with healthful drinks /** Dr. Rajat Trehan.

pages cm

ISBN 13: 978-93-340-7890-9    ISBN 10: 93-340-7890-1

1. Beverages--Health aspects. 2. Detoxification (Health) 3. Cooking, Indic. 4. Cookbooks. lcgft I. Heal Ur Body (Clinic : New Delhi, India), publisher. II. Title.

LCC TX815.T74 2024 | DDC 641.26 23

Dedicated to the cherished memory of my dearly departed parents, the late P.J. Trehan and the late Jyoti Trehan.

In their enduring love, relentless dedication, and profound commitment, I find the guiding light that has shaped the person I am today.

May their legacy of love and resilience continue to inspire and guide me on life's journey

# Disclaimer

This book provides information for reference purposes only and does not intend to replace or substitute professional medical advice. The author, the publisher, or any person directly or indirectly contributing to the publication or information disclaims any legal claims, express or implied. The information in this book is not a substitute for expert and professional medical advice. The author, publisher, and contributors assume no responsibility for any loss or damage caused, or allegedly caused, directly or indirectly by the use of the information contained in this book. The author and publisher expressly disclaim any liability incurred from the use or application of the contents of this book.

# Acknowledgements

I am extending my deepest and most heartfelt appreciation to the memory of my father, P.J. Trehan, and my mother, Jyoti Trehan, whose influence and legacy continue to inspire me. Their unwavering dedication to my upbringing and tireless efforts to instil in me a strong, rich cultural foundation have shaped my character and the very essence of this book. The values, principles, and wisdom they imparted to me during their lifetimes have remained with me, serving as a guiding force in both my personal life and creative endeavours. Though they are no longer physically present, their love, teachings, and profound influence have been a constant source of strength and inspiration as I embarked on this project. I owe them an immeasurable debt of gratitude for everything they gave me during the time we spent together. Their spirit continues to live on in the pages of this book, and I dedicate this work to their memory.

In addition to honouring my parents, I would like to offer a special acknowledgement to my brother, Dr Rajeev Trehan, who is a highly accomplished Cardiovascular and Thoracic Surgeon (CVTS), and his wife, Dr Meena Trehan, a skilled cardiac anaesthetist. Their unwavering support throughout this journey has been invaluable. The expertise, care, and dedication they bring to their own demanding professions have been a source of immense inspiration to me. Despite their busy lives, they have always found time to offer encouragement and advice, playing an essential role in the completion of this book. Their belief in this project and their constant motivation have given me the strength to keep moving forward, even during the most challenging times. I am deeply thankful for their presence and contributions, which have been vital in bringing "Irresistible Detox Elixirs" to life.

I also express my profound gratitude to my dedicated office staff, whose tireless efforts and commitment to this project have been nothing short of extraordinary. Beyond offering their unwavering support during the writing process, they took on the monumental task of typing the entire manuscript, ensuring that every detail was meticulously attended to. Their diligence, patience, and attention to detail were instrumental in turning this vision into a reality. They worked long hours, often going beyond the call of duty, to ensure that everything was in perfect order. Their hard work, dedication, and meticulous care have left an indelible mark on this book, and I am deeply appreciative of their efforts. Their contributions were essential in transforming my ideas into the finished manuscript, and their support has been invaluable throughout this journey.

In addition, I would like to acknowledge the invaluable assistance of Mr. Shhalaj Mittaal, Director of Shhalaj Publishing House, whose expertise in editing and formatting has been critical to bringing this book to its polished form. His meticulous attention to detail and professional insights ensured that every aspect of the text was refined to the highest standard. His dedication to excellence, coupled with his keen editorial eye, played a pivotal role in shaping the final version of this book. I am immensely grateful for his involvement and the care and precision he brought to the project. His expertise and guidance have been instrumental in elevating the quality of this work, and I sincerely appreciate his contributions to making this book the best it can be.

Finally, I would like to extend my heartfelt thanks to the many individuals who, over the course of my life and this project, have offered their insights, suggestions, and support. Whether through their knowledge of detox elixirs, their shared experiences, or simply their presence and encouragement, each person has contributed something valuable to this journey. Their insights and perspectives have added depth, richness, and diversity to "Irresistible Detox Elixirs," and their influence can be felt throughout the pages of this book. Each interaction, no matter how brief, has left an imprint on this project, and I am deeply grateful to all those who have shared their wisdom and experiences with me. Your contributions have enriched this work in ways that cannot be fully measured, and I am thankful for the impact you have had.

This journey has been a deeply personal and transformative one, and it would not have been possible without the involvement of each and every one of these individuals. I am profoundly grateful for the support, encouragement, and contributions of all who have been a part of this process. Whether directly or indirectly, you have all helped to bring this book to life, and for that, I am truly thankful. Your presence in my life and this project has been invaluable, and I am honoured to have had your support as I brought "Irresistible Detox Elixirs" to fruition. Thank you for being an integral part of this meaningful and rewarding venture. This book stands as a testament to your contributions, and I am forever grateful.

# Introduction

Welcome to the enchanting world of "Irresistible Detox Elixir," a comprehensive exploration into the realm of rejuvenating smoothies crafted to invigorate your body and tantalize your taste buds. In the fast-paced rhythm of modern life, this book stands as a haven, offering a treasure trove of wholesome ingredients and captivating elixirs that promise to cleanse, nourish, and elevate your well-being.

Within these pages, you'll embark on a sensory journey, discovering an array of irresistible detox elixirs meticulously designed to entice and transform. Bid farewell to the mundane and immerse yourself in the art of blending, where every sip is a symphony of flavours, a dance of nutrients, and a celebration of vitality.

The book "Irresistible Detox Elixir" goes beyond the ordinary, presenting a collection of elixirs that are not just recipes but experiences—a fusion of taste and wellness. From vibrant greens to luscious fruits, each concoction is a vibrant expression of health and indulgence. Let the late-night cravings be replaced with the desire for a refreshing elixir that not only satisfies the palate but also revitalizes the body.

As you leaf through these pages, be prepared to embrace a new chapter in your wellness journey. Elevate your mornings, boost your afternoons, and unwind in the evenings with elixirs that promise not just detoxification but a holistic embrace of vitality. The journey begins here, where each blend is a step towards a healthier, more vibrant you. Get ready to succumb to the allure of the "Irresistible Detox Elixir" and unlock the secrets to become a revitalized, irresistible you.

# Contents

# 1

# Phyto Green Detox Smoothie

Step into the world of vitality with the Phyto Green Detox Smoothie, a nutrient-packed elixir crafted from an assortment of green vegetables, fruits, and plant-based wonders. Tailored to deliver an intense infusion of vitamins, minerals, antioxidants, and phytonutrients, this smoothie is a dedicated companion on your journey to detoxification and overall well-being. Uncover the simplicity of the recipe, its invigorating method, and the myriad benefits it brings to your health.

**Ingredients:**

- 1 cup spinach (washed)
- 1 cup kale (washed and stems removed)
- 1 cucumber (peeled and chopped)
- 1 green apple (cored and chopped)
- 1 lemon (juiced)
- 1-inch piece of ginger (peeled)
- 1 cup coconut water or plain water
- Ice cubes (optional)

**Method of Preparation:**

- Wash all vegetables and fruits thoroughly.
- Peel and chop cucumber, core and chop green apple, and peel ginger.
- In a blender, combine spinach, kale, cucumber, green apple, ginger, and the lemon juice.

- Pour in one cup of coconut or plain water to facilitate blending.
- Blend until a smooth consistency is achieved. Adjust thickness by adding more water if needed.
- Add ice cubes to the blender and blend briefly to chill the juice.
- Pour the Phyto Green Detox Smoothie into a glass and relish the refreshing goodness!

**Benefits:**

**Detoxification:** Being rich in antioxidants, the blend supports the body's detoxification process by neutralizing harmful free radicals.

**Alkalizing Properties:** Green veggies contribute in balancing pH levels and reducing acidity in the body.

**Nutrient-rich:** Packed with essential vitamins and minerals for overall health and well-being.

**Digestive Health:** Fibre content aids in healthy digestion and regular bowel movements.

**Hydration:** Coconut water and the water content in fruits and veggies keep you well-hydrated.

**Immune Support:** Vitamin C from lemon and antioxidants bolster the immune system.

**Weight Management:** Low in calories, the smoothie aids in weight management when part of a balanced lifestyle.

Here's a vibrant and wholesome journey with the Phyto Green Detox Smoothie—sip, savour, and revitalize!

# 2

# Green Cleansing Detox Smoothie

A green cleansing detox is a dietary approach that involves consuming various nutrient-dense green foods and beverages to support the body's natural detoxification processes and promote overall health. The idea behind green cleansing detox is to provide the body with a rich source of vitamins, minerals, antioxidants and phytonutrients, which can aid in eliminating toxins and reducing inflammation. Here are some standard components and potential benefits of a green cleansing detox:

**Ingredients:**

**Green Vegetables:** Leafy greens like spinach, kale, chard, and arugula are rich in chlorophyll, which can aid in detoxifying the body and supporting liver function.

**Green Fruits:** Green apples, kiwis, and avocados are commonly included in green detox diets for their nutrient content and fibre.

**Herbs:** Herbs like parsley, cilantro, and mint may be incorporated for their detoxifying properties and fresh flavour.

**Citrus Fruits:** Lemons, limes, and oranges are often added to green detox drinks for their high vitamin C content and alkalizing effects.

**Green Smoothies/Juices:** Blending or juicing green vegetables and fruits can create nutrient-dense drinks that are easy to consume and digest.

**Green Tea:** Green tea is rich in antioxidants and can provide additional benefits for detoxification and overall health.

**Method of Preparation:**

- Gather your chosen greens, fruits, herbs, and green tea.
- Wash the ingredients thoroughly to ensure cleanliness.
- Combine the greens, fruits, herbs, and green tea in a blender.
- Blend until you get a smooth and vibrant green cleansing detox smoothie.
- Pour the detox smoothie into a glass and savour the health-boosting benefits of your homemade green elixir.

**Benefits of Green Cleansing Detox**

**Detoxification:** The abundance of antioxidants and phytonutrients in green foods can aid the body's natural detoxification by neutralizing free radicals and supporting liver function.

**Improves Digestion:** Green foods are typically fibre-rich, supporting healthy digestion and regular bowel movements.

**Increases Energy:** The nutrient density of green foods can provide a natural boost of energy and vitality.

**Reduces Inflammation:** Some components of green foods, such as chlorophyll and certain antioxidants, have anti-inflammatory properties, which can help reduce inflammation in the body.

**Weight Management:** Green cleansing detox, balanced diets, and exercise can contribute to weight management and healthy weight loss.

**Enhances Immune Function:** The high vitamin C content from citrus fruits and other nutrients in green foods can help strengthen the immune system.

**Alkalizing Effects:** Green foods are often alkaline-forming, which may help balance the body's pH levels and reduce acidity.

*Cheers to a flavourful and healthful journey!*

# 3

# Immune Booster Detox Smoothie

In the quest for a resilient and robust immune system, the "Immune Booster Detox" emerges as a potent elixir, carefully crafted with ingredients known for their immune-boosting properties. This simple, yet powerful smoothie, is a celebration of natural elements that can fortify your body's defences.

**Ingredients:**

**Fresh Ginger:** Ginger has anti-inflammatory properties and helps boost the immune system.

**Fresh Turmeric:** Turmeric contains curcumin, which has antioxidant and anti-inflammatory properties.

**Lemon or Lime:** Rich in vitamin C, which is known to support the immune system.

**Raw Honey:** Some studies suggest that raw honey has antibacterial and antioxidant properties. However, avoid giving honey to children under one year old.

**Water:** Hydration is essential for overall health, including the immune system.

**Method of preparation**

- Peel and chop a small piece of fresh ginger and fresh turmeric.
- Squeeze the juice from one lemon or lime.
- Heat water to a comfortable drinking temperature (not boiling).

- In a mug, mix the ginger, turmeric, lemon/lime juice, and add a teaspoon of raw honey (adjust to taste).
- Pour the heated water over the ingredients in the mug.
- Stir well and let the flavours steep for a few minutes.
- Remove the ginger and turmeric pieces if not desired.
- Savour the warm elixir and let it fortify your immune resilience.

**Benefits:**

**Ginger's Anti-Inflammatory Power:** Fresh ginger, a cornerstone of this detox, boasts anti-inflammatory properties. Known to soothe and support, ginger contributes to a strengthened immune system.

**Turmeric's Curcumin Kick:** Harnessing the power of curcumin, fresh turmeric lends its golden hue to the mix. This compound is renowned for its antioxidant and anti-inflammatory prowess, potentially enhancing immune response.

**Citrus Zing of Vitamin C:** A burst of citrus from lemon or lime brings more than just a zesty flavour. Laden with vitamin C, this ingredient is a well-known ally in supporting the immune system and overall health.

**Honey's Healing Touch:** Raw honey, with its potential antibacterial and antioxidant properties, sweetens the deal.

**Hydration for Health:** The base of this elixir is simple yet crucial—water. Adequate hydration is fundamental for overall health, and it plays a vital role in supporting the immune system.

*Cheers to a flavourful and healthful journey!*

# 4

## Berry Ginger Detox Smoothie

Embark on a delectable journey with the "Berry Ginger Detox," a vibrant fusion of antioxidant-rich blueberries, invigorating ginger, creamy avocado, and a touch of protein powder for a wholesome indulgence. This delightful concoction not only tantalizes your taste buds but also offers a myriad of benefits to support your overall well-being.

**Ingredients**

- Two cup frozen blueberries
- ½ inch ginger piece peeled, cut into slices
- 1 Avocado
- 1 tbsp protein powder
- 1 tbsp lemon juice
- 1 tbsp bee pollen
- Two cups of unsweetened almond milk.

**Instructions**

- Combine two cups of frozen blueberries,
- ½ inch sliced and peeled ginger,
- avocado, protein powder, lemon juice,
- One tablespoon of bee pollen, and
- Two cups of unsweetened almond milk in a blender.

Blend the ingredients thoroughly until you achieve a smooth and grand consistency. Enjoy this Berry Ginger Detox as a nutrient-packed, flavourful addition to your day.

**Benefits**

**Powerhouse of Antioxidants:** The frozen blueberries in this detox are bursting with antioxidants, which play a crucial role in neutralizing free radicals in the body. This antioxidant-rich blend may contribute to overall health and well-being.

**Anti-inflammatory Boost from Ginger:** The inclusion of ginger adds not only a zesty flavour but also anti-inflammatory properties. Ginger aids in reducing inflammation, providing potential benefits for joint health and overall bodily well-being.

**Creamy Nutrient Source of Avocado:** The addition of avocado introduces a creamy texture while providing a rich source of essential nutrients, including healthy monounsaturated fats, vitamins, and minerals. Avocado's nutritional profile may contribute to skin health and overall vitality.

**Protein Punch from Protein Powder:** A tablespoon of protein powder enhances the nutritional content, ensuring that your detox is not only delicious but also a source of protein. Protein is essential for repair and maintenance of muscles, making this detox a satisfying and nourishing option.

**Vitamin C Boost with Lemon:** One tablespoon of lemon not only adds a refreshing citrus twist but also contributes vitamin C, which is known for its immune-boosting properties, supporting your body's defence mechanisms.

**Bee Pollen for Nutrient Diversity:** Bee pollen is a nutrient-rich addition that brings a touch of sweetness to the mix. It contains a variety of vitamins, minerals, and antioxidants, potentially offering diverse health benefits.

**Nutrient-Rich Almond Milk Base:** The use of unsweetened almond milk not only ensures a smooth consistency but also adds a dose of nutrients. Almond milk is often fortified with vitamins like vitamin D and may contribute to bone health.

*Cheers to a flavourful and healthful journey!*

# 5

# Blood Red Detox Smoothie

Embark on a journey of vibrant health with our enticing "Blood Red Detox." This invigorating concoction not only captivates with its rich colour but also promises a symphony of benefits for your well-being. Let's explore the delightful combination of ingredients that make this detox a nourishing elixir.

**Ingredients:**

**Watermelon:** Bursting with hydration and a sweet flavour, watermelon forms the base of this detox, providing a refreshing and nutrient-packed foundation.

**Carrot:** Known for its vibrant orange hue, carrots contribute beta-carotene and other essential nutrients, promoting skin health and overall vitality.

**Cranberries:** These tart berries add a delightful tang to the mix while bringing antioxidant properties that may support a healthy immune system.

**Pomegranates:** Packed with antioxidants and a distinctive sweetness, pomegranates lend their unique flavour and potential anti-inflammatory benefits to the detox.

**Strawberries:** Not only do strawberries contribute to the drink's appealing red hue, but they also bring a dose of vitamin C and other antioxidants.

**Instructions**

- Begin by peeling the watermelon, pomegranate, and carrot.

- Thoroughly wash all the ingredients to ensure cleanliness and optimal flavour.
- Place the peeled and cleaned watermelon, carrot, cranberries, pomegranates, and strawberries in a blender or "grinder."
- Blend the ingredients until a smooth and luscious juice is extracted.

**Benefits**

**Aids in Weight Loss:** The nutrient-rich content of this detox, coupled with its hydrating nature, supports weight loss as part of a balanced diet and healthy lifestyle.

**Improves Skin Health:** The combination of beta-carotene from carrots and antioxidants from berries contributes to a radiant complexion and overall skin well-being.

**Boosts Immunity:** Cranberries and pomegranates bring a burst of antioxidants that enhance your body's defence mechanisms and support a robust immune system.

**Cures Inflammation:** The anti-inflammatory properties inherent in the ingredients, particularly in cranberries and pomegranates, aid in alleviating inflammation.

**Keeps Eyes Healthy:** The presence of vitamin A from carrots contributes to eye health, promoting good vision and overall ocular well-being.

Incorporate this Blood Red Detox into your routine for a flavourful and health-boosting experience. Sip your way to wellness and relish the benefits that this vibrant elixir can bring to your life.

*Cheers to a flavourful and healthy journey!*

# 6

# Ginger Explosion Detox

Prepare to awaken your senses with the invigorating "Ginger Explosion Detox." This simple yet powerful elixir is not just a burst of flavour; it's a wellness potion crafted around the potent properties of ginger. Join us on a journey that fuses simplicity and efficacy for a refreshing and beneficial experience.

### Ingredients

**Grated Ginger:** The star of the show, ginger, isn't just a spice; it's a treasure trove of antioxidants. Embrace its natural goodness as it takes centre stage in this detox, bringing a delightful explosion of flavour and health benefits.

**Normal Water:** A humble yet essential component, normal water serves as the canvas for this ginger-infused masterpiece. Stay hydrated while relishing the simplicity of this rejuvenating beverage.

### Method of Preparation

**Grated Ginger:** Begin by grating a generous amount of fresh ginger, unlocking its aromatic and therapeutic essence.

**Normal Water:** Combine the grated ginger with normal water, creating a harmonious blend that promises both hydration and a flavourful kick.

**Boiling on Low Heat:** Gently simmer the mixture on low heat for approximately five minutes, allowing the ginger to infuse its essence into the water.

**Benefits**

**Antioxidant Richness:** The ginger in this detox is a powerhouse of antioxidants, aiding in combating oxidative stress and promoting overall cellular health.

**Digestive Harmony:** Experience relief from gas and constipation as ginger's natural properties work to soothe and regulate the digestive system.

**Weight Management Support:** Incorporating ginger into your routine may contribute to weight loss efforts, making this detox not only a treat for your taste buds but also a potential ally in your wellness journey.

As you indulge in the "Ginger Explosion Detox," savour the fusion of simplicity and health benefits. Let this elixir be a daily ritual, a burst of goodness that not only delights your palate but also nurtures your body from the inside out.

*Cheers to a flavourful and healthful journey!*

# 7

# Orange, Carrot, Ginger Detox

Embark on a journey of vibrant rejuvenation with the "Orange, Carrot, Ginger Detox." This refreshing elixir isn't just a symphony of flavours; it's a harmonious blend of nutrients that nourish and invigorate. Join us as we explore the goodness of oranges, carrots, and ginger, crafting a detox that not only tantalizes your taste buds but also bestows a myriad of health benefits.

**Ingredients**

**Large Carrot:** Packed with nutrients, carrots aren't just good for your eyes; they contribute to radiant skin and support weight loss and digestion.

**Oranges:** Bursting with nutrients, antioxidants, and immune-boosting properties, oranges add a citrusy zing to this detox, elevating both flavour and well-being.

**Raw Turmeric (crushed):** This golden spice, in its raw form, introduces anti-inflammatory and antioxidant properties, enhancing the drink's health benefits.

**Ginger (crushed):** Ginger, a versatile root, lends its natural prowess to this elixir, aids in the relief of sore throat, digestion, bloating, and stomach cramps.

**Lemon (juiced):** The addition of lemon juice not only provides a refreshing acidity but also contributes to the detoxifying nature of this beverage.

**Method of Preparation**

Follow the simple steps in the preparation of the "Orange, Carrot, Ginger Detox".:

**Extract Juice:** Separate the juice of the orange and carrot, capturing the essence of their natural goodness.

**Blend Ginger and Turmeric:** In a blender, combine crushed ginger and turmeric, blending for 30 seconds to create a vibrant base for the detox.

**Add Lemon Juice:** Squeeze half a lemon into the blend, infusing a zesty kick that complements the other flavours.

**Filter and Serve:** After blending, filter the mixture to attain a smooth and luscious elixir. Serve and revel in the fusion of health and taste.

**Benefits**

**Nutrient-Rich Immunity Boost:** Oranges contribute a wealth of nutrients and antioxidants, enhancing your immune system's resilience.

**Skin Health and Weight Management:** Carrots, with their fibre content, promote healthy skin and aid in weight loss and digestion.

**Anti-inflammatory Support:** Raw turmeric and ginger bring anti-inflammatory benefits, offering relief from various ailments, including sore throat and bloating.

Savour the "Orange, Carrot, Ginger Detox" as more than just a beverage – let it be a ritual that uplifts your spirits and nurtures your well-being.

*Cheers to a flavourful and healthy journey!*

# 8

# Antioxidant Detox Drink

Embark on a journey of well-being with the enticing blend of flavours in the "Antioxidant Detox Drink." This harmonious concoction not only delights your taste buds but also celebrates the healthful synergy of nature's antioxidant-rich treasures.

**Ingredients:**

**Lemon:** Infused with vitamin C, lemon adds a citrusy zing and a powerful dose of antioxidants to the mix.

**Ginger:** This versatile root enhances the drink with its anti-inflammatory and antioxidant properties, elevating its overall health benefits.

**Apple:** Offering natural sweetness and a variety of antioxidants, apples contribute to the overall well-being of the drink.

**Mint:** Known for its refreshing flavour, mint introduces a delightful twist while adding to the antioxidant content of the concoction.

**Waterlemon:** Hydrating and sweet, watermelon complements the detox, contributing to both flavour and healthful properties.

**Cucumber:** Low in calories and high in antioxidants, cucumber enhances the drink with refreshing and hydrating qualities.

**Cranberry:** Rich in antioxidants, cranberries bring both flavour and health benefits to the vibrant mix.

**Grapefruit:** Enhancing taste and contributing to eye health, grapefruit is a citrusy addition with overall well-being benefits.

**Dandelion:** Adding to the antioxidant richness, dandelion introduces potential detoxifying properties to the blend.

**Method:**

To prepare this antioxidant-rich elixir, follow these simple steps:

**Prepare Ingredients:** Mix lemon juice, mint, apple, watermelon, cucumber, cranberry, grapefruit, dandelion, and grated ginger.

**Combine and Grind:** Blend all the ingredients together to form a vibrant and flavourful concoction.

**Enjoy the Antioxidant Detox:** Savour the goodness as you sip on this revitalizing elixir, letting the antioxidants invigorate your body and uplift your sense of well-being.

**Benefits:**

**Reduction of Oxidative Stress:** The antioxidants in this drink work together to reduce oxidative stress, safeguarding your cells and promoting overall health.

**Support for Disease Prevention:** Antioxidants play a pivotal role in disease prevention by neutralizing free radicals that could contribute to various health issues.

**Enhancement of Eye Health:** Ingredients like lemon and grapefruit contribute to supporting eye health, aiding in maintaining optimal vision.

**Boost to Brain Function:** The antioxidants present in the detox aid in enhancing brain function, supporting cognitive health and mental clarity.

**Improvement in Mental Health:** This detox contributes in improving mental health, offering a refreshing and nourishing experience for your mind.

**Reduction of Inflammation:** The potent anti-inflammatory properties of these ingredients synergize to reduce inflammation in the body.

**Support for Healthy Ageing:** Embrace the natural ageing process with grace, as the antioxidants in this drink contribute to healthy ageing, promoting longevity and vitality.

Make the "Antioxidant Detox Drink" a cherished part of your daily ritual, revelling in the fusion of health and taste.

*Here's to your vibrant and nourished self!*

# 9

# Lemon Tulsi Detox

Embark on a journey of holistic well-being with the "Lemon Tulsi Detox." This revitalizing concoction transcends the ordinary, blends the aromatic essence of tulsi, the zesty twist of lemon, and the soothing warmth of ginger. Elevate your tea experience as we delve into a beverage that not only tantalizes your taste buds but also bestows a multitude of health benefits.

**Ingredients:**

**Tulsi (10-15 leaves):** This sacred herb, also known as holy basil, infuses the detox with its aromatic and therapeutic properties, offering a symphony of flavours and health benefits.

**Grated Ginger (one tsp):** Ginger, with its anti-inflammatory and digestive properties, adds a touch of warmth and well-being to the concoction.

**Tea powder (one tsp):** Black tea, rich in antioxidants, forms the base of this detox, contributing to overall health benefits.

**Jaggery (one tsp):** Natural sweetness from jaggery not only enhances the flavour but also provides essential minerals, offering a healthier alternative to refined sugar.

**Lemon Juice (one tsp):** The addition of lemon juice not only brings a refreshing citrusy note but also provides a dose of vitamin C, boosting immunity.

**Black Salt (A pinch):** A pinch of black salt not only enhances the taste but also adds minerals, aiding in digestion and promoting electrolyte balance.

**Black Peppercorns (one tsp):** Adding a hint of spice, black peppercorns contribute flavour and possess anti-inflammatory and digestive properties.

**Method: of Preparation**

To prepare the "Lemon Tulsi Detox," follow these simple steps:

**Combine Ingredients:** In a deep pan, bring together tulsi leaves, black pepper, and grated ginger with two cups of water.

**Boil on Low Heat:** Simmer the mixture on low heat for ten minutes, allowing the flavours to meld and infuse into the water.

**Add Tea Powder:** Add tea powder and remove the mixture from heat.

**Cover and add Jaggery:** Cover the pan for two minutes, allowing the jaggery to dissolve and sweeten the concoction.

**Strain and Season:** Strain the liquid and add a pinch of black salt and lemon juice, balancing the flavours and enhancing the detoxifying properties.

**Serve Immediately:** Pour into a cup and savour the rejuvenating blend immediately, letting its warmth and goodness envelop you.

**Benefits:**

**Relief for Sore Throat:** The combination of tulsi, ginger, and lemon provides relief for a sore throat, offering comfort during cold seasons.

**Digestive Support:** Ginger, black salt, and jaggery collectively contribute to maintain digestive health, ensuring your system stays on track.

**Cold Comfort:** With its soothing properties, this detox brings relief even if you're battling a cold, providing a comforting experience.

Experience the "Lemon Tulsi Detox" as more than a tea—it's a mindful ritual that nurtures your body and soul. Embrace the goodness and elevate your well-being with every sip.

# 10

## Cilantro Fiesta Drink

Embark on a flavour-filled fiesta for your senses with the "Cilantro Fiesta Drink." This vibrant concoction is a celebration of the zesty freshness of cilantro, harmoniously blended with complementary ingredients to create a beverage that not only tantalizes your taste buds but also promises a plethora of health benefits.

**Ingredients:**

**Cilantro (Coriander leaves):** The star of this fiesta, cilantro, brings its distinct and refreshing flavour along with potential health benefits, including antioxidants and digestive support.

**Cucumber:** Adding a crisp and hydrating element, cucumber not only enhances the drink's texture but also contributes to overall hydration and skin health.

**Lime or Lemon Juice:** Infusing a citrusy kick, lime or lemon juice adds a tangy flavour and provides a burst of vitamin C, supporting immunity.

**Green Apple:** Offering a subtle sweetness and a host of vitamins, green apple complements the cilantro, creating a well-rounded and refreshing profile.

**Ginger:** Known for its anti-inflammatory properties, ginger adds warmth to the fiesta while contributing to digestive health.

**Black Salt:** A pinch of black salt not only enhances the overall taste but also provides essential minerals, aiding digestion and electrolyte balance.

**Chilled Water:** Serving as the base, chilled water brings all the ingredients together, ensuring a crisp and refreshing finish.

**Method of preparation:**

To craft the "Cilantro Fiesta Drink," follow these simple steps:

**Prepare Ingredients:** Gather fresh cilantro, cucumber slices, lime or lemon juice, diced green apple, grated ginger, and a pinch of black salt.

**Blend Together:** In a blender, mix all the ingredients with chilled water, creating a vibrant and invigorating concoction.

**Blend Until Smooth:** Blend the ingredients until smooth, ensuring a harmonious fusion of flavours and a refreshing consistency.

**Strain (Optional):** If needed, strain the liquid to achieve a smoother texture.

**Serve Chilled:** Pour the Cilantro Fiesta Drink into glasses over ice, serving immediately to relish its crisp and revitalizing essence.

**Benefits:**

**Antioxidant Boost:** Cilantro, green apple, and citrus juice contribute to the drink's antioxidant content, promoting cellular health and combating oxidative stress.

**Hydration Support:** Cucumber and chilled water ensure optimal hydration, essential for overall well-being and skin health.

**Digestive Harmony:** Ginger and black salt collectively aid in digestion, promoting a healthy gut and digestive system.

**Vitamin Infusion:** Lime or lemon juice and green apple introduce a treasure of vitamins, particularly vitamin C, supporting immunity and overall vitality.

**Refreshing and Revitalizing:** The crisp and zesty nature of this drink provides a refreshing experience, making it an ideal choice to revitalize your senses.

Embrace the fiesta of flavours and benefits with the "Cilantro Fiesta Drink," a delightful addition to your wellness routine that promises both healthful and indulgent satisfaction.

*Cheers to vibrant well-being!*

# 11

## Pineapple and Cabbage Juice

Immerse yourself in a refreshing journey with the "Pineapple and Cabbage Juice," a vibrant concoction that merges the tropical sweetness of pineapple with the crispness of cabbage. Beyond its tantalizing taste, this juice is a hydrating and diuretic elixir, offering not only a flavourful experience but also contributing to weight loss goals.

**Ingredients:**

**Cold Water (100 ml):** A hydrating base, cold water forms the foundation of this juice, ensuring a crisp and refreshing finish.

**Cucumber Slice:** Adds a mild and hydrating element, a slice of cucumber complements the overall texture and enhances the juice's hydrating properties.

**Green Apple with Peel:** Infusing a subtle sweetness, green apple, along with its peel, contributes to the juice's flavour profile while providing vitamins and fibre.

**Pineapple Slice:** The star of the show, pineapple brings its tropical sweetness and natural enzymes, by adding a delightful twist to the juice.

**Grated Ginger (one teaspoon):** This warming spice not only enhances the flavour but also contributes to digestion and potential anti-inflammatory benefits.

**Chia Seeds (one teaspoon):** Packed with nutrients, chia seeds add a touch of crunch while providing omega-3 fatty acids, fibre, and antioxidants.

**Cabbage Leaf:** A unique addition, cabbage brings a refreshing and mild flavour, contributing to the juice's hydrating and weight loss properties.

**Method of Preparation**

To create the "Pineapple and Cabbage Juice," follow these simple steps:

**Combine Ingredients:** In a blender, blend cold water, cucumber, green apple with peel, pineapple slice, grated ginger, chia seeds, and a cabbage leaf until well combined.

**Strain and Drink:** Strain the mixture to achieve a smooth consistency, and drink the juice, preferably without sweetener.

**Storage:** This juice can be stored in a well-sealed container in the refrigerator for up to six hours.

**Benefits:**

**Supports Weight Loss:** With its rich water content and diuretic properties, this juice becomes an excellent addition to a weight loss diet, containing about 156 calories per 250 mL serving.

**Boosts Hydration:** The combination of ingredients, particularly cucumber, pineapple, and cabbage, ensures optimal hydration, supporting overall well-being.

**Nutrient-Rich:** Green apples, chia seeds, and cabbage contribute essential nutrients such as vitamins, fibre, and antioxidants, enhancing the nutritional profile of the juice.

**Aids Digestion:** The presence of grated ginger and the fibre from apple and cabbage collectively aids digestion, promoting a healthy gut.

Sip and savour the goodness of the "Pineapple and Cabbage Juice," a hydrating and flavourful companion on your journey to wellness.

*Cheers to a refreshing and healthful indulgence!*

# 12

# Pomegranate, Beet and Aloe Power Detox

Elevate your well-being with the invigorating blend of the "Pomegranate, Beet and Aloe Power Detox," a concoction designed to deliver a burst of freshness and health benefits. Immerse yourself in the synergy of sweetness of pomegranate, earthy richness of beetroot, and the soothing essence of aloe vera. Beyond its tantalizing taste, this power detox aims to address constipation, regulate blood pressure, boost immunity, and lower cholesterol levels.

**Ingredients:**

**Fresh Aloe Vera Leaf:** Harness the therapeutic properties of aloe vera by extracting its gel from a fresh leaf, ensuring a clean and revitalizing addition to the detox.

**Beetroot (1/2 cup, chopped):** Infuse the detox with the earthy sweetness of beetroot, which provides not only flavour but also essential nutrients and potential blood pressure-regulating benefits.

**Pomegranate Juice or Amla Juice (2 cups):** Embrace the antioxidant-rich goodness of pomegranate or amla (Indian gooseberry) juice, offering a burst of sweetness and immune-boosting properties.

**Black Pepper Powder (1/4 tsp):** Introduce a hint of warmth and spice with black pepper, contributing not only to flavour but also potentially aiding digestion.

**Method of Preparation:**

To create the "Pomegranate, Beet & Aloe Power Detox," follow these simple steps:

**Preparation of Aloe Vera Gel:** Remove the outer layer of the aloe vera leaf, extract its gel, and clean it thoroughly for a pristine addition to the detox.

**Blend Pomegranate Juice and Beetroot:** In a blender, combine pomegranate juice and chopped beetroot. Blend smoothly to create a vibrant and flavourful base.

**Add Aloe Vera Gel:** Incorporate the aloe vera gel into the blend, giving it a whiz to ensure a smooth and well-combined mixture.

**Introduce Black Pepper:** Finally, add black pepper to the mix, enhancing the detox with a touch of warmth.

**Serve:** Pour the "Pomegranate, Beet & Aloe Power Detox" into a glass and relish the invigorating fusion of flavours and health benefits.

**Benefits:**

**Relief from Constipation:** The combination of aloe vera, pomegranate, and beet aims to address constipation, promoting digestive health.

**Blood Pressure Regulation:** Beetroot, known for its potential blood pressure-lowering effects, contributes in maintaining cardiovascular health.

**Boost Immunity:** Pomegranate and aloe vera are packed with antioxidants, providing a substantial boost to the immune system.

**Cholesterol Level Management:** The detox, with its combination of ingredients, may aid in managing cholesterol levels and promoting heart health.

Savour the rejuvenating essence of the "Pomegranate, Beet & Aloe Power Detox" as it becomes a flavourful and healthful addition to your wellness routine.

*Cheers to a vibrant and nourished you!*

# 13

## Honey Lemon Ginger Tea

Indulge in the comforting embrace of the "Honey Lemon Ginger Tea," a soothing elixir designed not only to warm your senses but also to provide a potent boost to your immune system. Immerse yourself in the invigorating combination of ginger's spiciness, the citrusy zing of lemon, and the natural sweetness of honey. Apart from its delightful flavour, this tea unfolds as a compelling antibiotic, fosters immune strength and potentially inhibits the development and spread of disease cells.

**Ingredients:**

**Water (2 Cups):** A comforting base, water serves as the canvas for this tea, offering hydration and a soothing foundation.

**Ginger (1 tsp, finely chopped):** Infuse the tea with the spiciness of finely chopped ginger, known for its anti-inflammatory and immune-boosting properties.

**Tea Leaves (1 tsp for every cup):** Choose your preferred tea leaves, whether black, green, or herbal, to add depth and richness to the flavour profile.

**Lemon Juice (1 tsp):** Introduce a burst of citrusy freshness with lemon juice, rich in bioflavonoids that may support immunity and combat the development of disease cells.

**Honey (1 tsp):** Elevate the natural sweetness with honey, which adds not only flavour but potential antibacterial and soothing qualities also.

**Method of preparation:**

To prepare the "Honey Lemon Ginger Tea," follow these simple steps:

**Boil Water with Ginger:** In a pan, boil two cups of water, add finely chopped ginger to infuse its spiciness into the liquid.

**Add Tea Leaves, Lemon, and Honey:** Once the water begins to boil, introduce tea leaves, lemon juice, and honey, allowing the tea to simmer for some time to absorb the flavours.

**Let the Tea Simmer:** Allow the tea to simmer, letting the amalgamation of ingredients unfold, enhancing both flavour and potential health benefits.

**Filter the Tea:**Switch off the flame and remove the tea from the stove. Filter the tea to remove the tea leaves and ginger, ensuring a smooth and delightful consistency.

**Serve:** Pour the 'Honey Lemon Ginger Tea' into a cup, savour the comforting aroma and embrace the immune-boosting warmth.

**Benefits:**

**Boost Immune System:** Ginger, lemon, and honey collectively contribute to boosting the immune system, providing resilience against colds and influenza.

**Antibiotic Properties:** This tea unfolds as a compelling antibiotic, potentially aiding in combating infections and supporting overall health.

**Bioflavonoid Support:** The bioflavonoids in lemons help prevent the development, spread, and potential formation of cancer cells.

Relish the therapeutic warmth and flavour of the "Honey Lemon Ginger Tea," making it a cherished part of your routine for both comfort and well-being.

*Here's to healthful sipping!*

# 14

## Ginger Litchi Lemonade Detox

Immerse yourself in the refreshing allure of the "Ginger Litchi Lemonade Detox," a revitalizing elixir that not only quenches your thirst but also delivers a host of health benefits. Indulge in the invigorating fusion of minced ginger, zesty lemon juice, and the luscious sweetness of lychee. This detox not only aids in weight reduction but also boosts digestive power, strengthens immunity, and offers relief from migraine.

**Ingredients:**

**Ginger (1/2 Cup, minced):** Infuse the detox with the spiciness of minced ginger, known for its digestion-boosting and metabolism-enhancing properties.

**Fresh Lemon Juice (1/2 Cup):** Add a burst of citrusy freshness with fresh lemon juice, providing vitamin C and a tangy twist to the detox.

**Ice Cubes (as needed):** Enhance the refreshing quality of the detox by adding ice cubes to achieve the perfect chill.

**Lychee Juice (one glass):** Embrace the exotic sweetness of lychee juice, offering a delightful and hydrating base for the detox.

**Grapes (one cup, chopped):** Introduce a burst of natural sweetness and antioxidants with chopped grapes, enhancing both the flavour and nutritional content.

**Chia Seeds (1/2 cup):** Boost the detox with the nutritional powerhouse of chia seeds, providing omega-3 fatty acids, fibre, and additional texture.

**Mint Leaves:** Elevate the freshness of the detox with mint leaves, offering a cooling and aromatic element to the concoction.

**A Pinch of Salt:** Add a pinch of salt to balance the flavours and enhance the overall taste of the detox.

**Method of preparation:**

To prepare the "Ginger Litchi Lemonade Detox," follow these simple steps:

**Combine Ginger, Lemon Juice, and Lychee Juice:** In a jar, mix minced ginger, fresh lemon juice, and lychee juice, creating the flavourful foundation of the detox.

**Add Ice and Salt:** Introduce ice cubes for a refreshing chill, and add a pinch of salt to enhance the taste. Mix well to ensure even distribution.

**Include Chopped Grapes and Chia Seeds:** Add chopped grapes and chia seeds to the jar, infusing the detox with sweetness, antioxidants, and nutritional richness.

**Garnish with Mint Leaves:** After thorough mixing, garnish the detox with fresh mint leaves, elevating both the visual appeal and aromatic quality.

**Enjoy and Indulge:** Dive into the delightful experience of the "Ginger Litchi Lemonade Detox," savouring the harmonious blend of flavours and relishing the multitude of health benefits.

**Benefits:**

**Weight Reduction:** The detox aids in weight reduction, due to the metabolism-boosting properties of ginger and the hydrating quality of lychee.

**Increases Digestive Power:** Ginger contributes in enhancing digestive power, promoteing a healthy gut and efficient digestion.

**Immunity Strengthening:** The combination of lemon, lychee, and ginger works synergistically to strengthen the immune system, providing resilience against illnesses.

**Migraine Relief:** Enjoy relief from migraines, as ginger's anti-inflammatory properties help alleviate symptoms.

Delight in the healthful indulgence of the "Ginger Litchi Lemonade Detox," making it a refreshing and nourishing addition to your wellness routine.

*Cheers to vibrant health and delicious sipping!*

# 15

# Coconut Water with Lemon and Mint Detox

Embark on a journey of revitalization with the "Coconut Water with Lemon and Mint Detox," a refreshing elixir that not only quenches your thirst but also bestows a wealth of health benefits. Immerse yourself in the natural goodness of coconut water, complemented by the zesty twist of lemon, the sweetness of honey, and the invigorating freshness of mint. This detox is not only rich in vitamins and minerals but also acts as a preventive measure against dehydration, aids digestion, and provides a substantial dose of immune-boosting Vitamin C.

**Ingredients:**

**Coconut:** Utilize the hydrating treasure of a coconut, extract its water to form the refreshing base of the detox.

**Mint Leaves:** Infuse the detox with a burst of freshness and aroma by adding mint leaves, which contributes not only to flavour but also the potential digestive benefits.

**Honey (1 tbsp):** Elevate the sweetness naturally with honey, adding a touch of indulgence and potential antibacterial properties.

**Lemon:** Introduce the citrusy essence of lemon, which is a rich source of Vitamin C and provides a zesty flavour.

**Method of preparation:**

Follow these simple steps to prepare the tasty and healthy"Coconut Water with Lemon and Mint Detox," :

**Extract Coconut Water:** Take a coconut and extract its water into a glass, ensuring the hydrating foundation of the detox.

**Scrape Coconut Flesh:** With a spoon, scrape out the flesh of the coconut, cut it into fine pieces, and mix it into the coconut water for added texture and flavour.

**Add Lemon, Mint, Honey, and Lemon Juice:** Introduce lemon slices, mint leaves, a tablespoon of honey, and a squeeze of lemon juice into the mix, creating a harmonious blend of flavours.

**Mix Well:** Stir the ingredients well to ensure the even distribution of flavours and the infusion of all the healthful elements.

**Benefits:**

**Rich in Vitamins and Minerals:** Coconut water, lemon, and mint collectively contribute to the detox's richness in vitamins and minerals, promoting overall health.

**Prevents Dehydration:** The hydrating property of coconut water serve as a natural defence against dehydration, ensuring optimal fluid balance in the body.

**Aids in Digestion:** Mint leaves and lemon contribute to digestive benefits, potentially aiding in soothing the digestive system.

**Rich in Vitamin C:** Enjoy a substantial dose of immune-boosting Vitamin C from the addition of lemon, supporting your body's defence against illnesses.

Sip and savour the "Coconut Water with Lemon and Mint Detox," relishing both its delightful flavour and the healthful benefits it brings to your well-being.

*Here's to a refreshing and nourishing experience!*

# 16

## Aam Panna Detox

Celebrate the essence of summer with the "Aam Panna Detox," a refreshing elixir crafted from the beloved green mango. Beyond its delightful taste, Aam Panna stands as a seasonal favourite, not only for its deliciousness but also for its detoxifying benefits. As the mangoes grace the summer abundance, Aam Panna becomes a hydrating and detoxifying ally, protecting your body from dehydration and offering a rejuvenating experience.

**Ingredients:**

**Green Mangoes (500 gm):** Harness the vibrant flavours of green mangoes, a quintessential summer fruit, for the base of the detox.

**Sugar (1/2 cup):** Add sweetness to balance the tartness of the green mangoes, enhancing the overall taste of the Aam Panna.

**Salt (two tsp):** Introduce salt to enhance the flavours and provide electrolyte balance, a crucial element during the summer months.

**Kala Namak (Black Rock Salt, two tsp):** Infuse the detox with the distinctive taste of kala namak, contributing to both flavour and potential digestive benefits.

**Roasted and Powdered Cumin Seeds (2 tsp):** Elevate the aromatic profile with roasted and powdered cumin seeds, offering a touch of warmth and depth.

**Finely Chopped Mint Leaves (two Tbsp):** Add a burst of freshness with finely chopped mint leaves, providing a cooling and aromatic element.

**Water (two cups):** Form the hydrating base of the detox, ensuring a refreshing and revitalizing experience.

**Method of Preparation:**

Follow these simple steps in the preparation of "Aam Panna Detox".

**Boil Green Mangoes:** Boil 2 to 4 green mangoes until they are well-cooked. Once cooked, allow them to cool.

**Prepare the Detox Mixture:** In a glass of cold water, add sugar, salt, kala namak, roasted and powdered cumin seeds, and finely chopped mint leaves. Mix well with a spoon.

**Add Boiled Mango Pulp:** Once the boiled mangoes are cooled, extract their pulp and add it to the detox mixture in the glass.

**Include Ice Cubes:** Enhance the refreshing quality by adding 2 to 4 ice cubes to the glass, ensuring a chilled and invigorating experience.

**Mix and Enjoy:** Stir the contents well, allowing the flavours to meld, and then savour the Aam Panna Detox, relishing the taste of summer.

**Benefits:**

**Detoxifying Properties:** Aam Panna acts as a natural detox, refreshing your body and promoting overall well-being.

**Prevents Hydration and Dehydration:** With its hydrating base and the goodness of green mangoes, Aam Panna protects against dehydration during the hot summer months.

**Digestive Support:** The inclusion of kala namak and roasted cumin seeds may offer digestive benefits, contributing to a healthy digestive system.

Indulge in the season's bounty with the "Aam Panna Detox," a flavourful and healthful choice that captures the essence of summer in every sip.

*Here's to the joy of sipping and staying refreshed!*

# 17

## Detox Haldi Tea

Embark on a journey of wellness with the "Detox Haldi Tea," a harmonious blend of antioxidant-rich turmeric, immune-boosting ginger, and the warming essence of black pepper. Beyond its delightful flavour, this tea offers a perfect combination of ingredients with numerous health benefits. Turmeric, the star ingredient, takes centre stage as a potent liver-cleansing spice, contributing to improved liver function and enhanced immunity.

**Ingredients:**

**Haldi (Turmeric 1/2 tsp):** Embrace the golden goodness of turmeric, a powerful antioxidant and anti-inflammatory spice, forming the heart of the Detox Haldi Tea.

**Ginger (1/2 tsp, chopped):** Infuse the tea with the zesty and immune-boosting properties of ginger, adding depth and warmth to the flavour profile.

**Black Pepper (1/4 tsp):** Introduce a touch of spice with black pepper, not only enhancing the taste but also potentially aiding in the absorption of turmeric's beneficial compounds.

**Honey (one tsp):** Elevate the sweetness naturally with honey, offering not only a delightful taste but also potential antibacterial and soothing properties.

**Water (two cups):** Form the hydrating base of the tea, ensuring a comforting and healthful beverage.

**Method of preparation:**

To prepare the "Detox Haldi Tea," follow these simple steps:

**Heat Water:** Take a bowl, add water, and heat it until it reaches a simmer.

**Add Ingredients:** Once the water is simmering, add haldi (turmeric), chopped ginger, black pepper, and honey to the bowl, creating a rich and flavourful infusion.

**Stir Well:** Stir the ingredients well, ensuring the even distribution of flavours and the amalgamation of the healthful properties.

**Boil and Reduce:** Keep boiling the water until it reduces to half, allowing the flavours to intensify and the beneficial compounds to infuse into the tea.

**Serve Hot:** Once the tea is ready, serve it hot, embracing the soothing warmth and the potential health benefits.

**Benefits:**

**Antioxidant and Anti-Inflammatory Power:** The combination of turmeric, ginger, and black pepper delivers a powerful blend of antioxidants and anti-inflammatory ingredients, promoting overall well-being.

**Liver-Cleansing:** Turmeric's potent properties make it a valuable spice for liver cleansing, contributing to improved liver function.

**Immune Boost:** The immune-boosting qualities of turmeric and ginger collectively enhance the body's defences, supporting a robust immune system.

Indulge in the nourishing experience of the "Detox Haldi Tea," savouring the rich flavours and basking in the potential health benefits it brings to your wellness routine.

*Here's to a healthful sipping and a rejuvenated you!*

# 18

## Pink Salt Ginger Detox Water

Revitalize your senses and invigorate your well-being with the "Pink Salt Ginger Detox Water," a sweet and sour elixir crafted with the goodness of ginger, pink salt, and the optional touch of honey. Beyond its delightful taste, this detox water serves as a refreshing beverage, offering a harmonious blend of flavours to refresh your mind and soul.

**Ingredients:**

**Water (1 glass):** Form the hydrating base of the detox water, ensuring a refreshing and revitalizing experience.

**Pink Salt (A pinch):** Infuse the water with the mineral-rich essence of pink salt, adding depth to the flavour profile and potential electrolyte balance.

**Ginger (1/2 inch, grated):** Embrace the spiciness and health benefits of ginger, contributing both flavour and potential anti-inflammatory properties.

**Lemon Juice (1/2 lemon):** Introduce a burst of citrusy freshness with lemon juice, providing a zesty twist to the detox water.

**Honey (1 tsp, optional):** Add honey to enhance sweetness naturally, offering not only a delightful taste but also potential antibacterial and soothing properties.

**Method of Preparation:**

To prepare the "Pink Salt Ginger Detox Water," follow these simple steps:

**Boil Water with Grated Ginger:** Boil the water with grated ginger, allowing the flavours of ginger to infuse into the water. Strain the mixture into a glass.

**Cool Down:** Let the water cool down for a while, maintaining a warm or lukewarm temperature rather than turning it completely cold.

**Add Pink Salt, Lemon Juice, and Honey:** Once the water is cooled, add a pinch of pink salt, lemon juice, and honey (optional) to the glass, creating a balanced and flavourful concoction.

**Mix Well:** Stir the ingredients well, ensuring the even distribution of flavours and the infusion of all the healthful elements.

**Benefits:**

**Refreshment for Mind and Soul:** The combination of sweet and sour flavours in this detox water provides a refreshing experience, revitalizing both the mind and soul.

**Ginger's Health Benefits:** Ginger contributes not only to the flavour but also potential anti-inflammatory properties, promoting overall well-being.

**Pink Salt's Minerals:** Pink salt adds minerals to the water, potentially providing electrolyte balance and supporting hydration.

**Citrusy Zing with Lemon:** Lemon juice adds a burst of citrusy freshness, enriching the water with Vitamin C and a zesty twist.

Indulge in the rejuvenating experience of the "Pink Salt Ginger Detox Water," savouring the delightful fusion of flavours and embracing the potential health benefits it brings to your hydration routine.

*Here's to a refreshing and nourishing sip!*

# 19

# Jeera Water Detox

Unlock the simplicity of detoxification with "Jeera Detox Water," a refreshing elixir crafted from humble yet potent cumin seeds. Jeera, known for its distinct flavour and potential health benefits, takes centre stage in this detox water, offering an effortless and accessible way to promote overall well-being. Let the subtle spiciness of cumin seeds infuse into the water, creating a beverage that not only revitalizes but may also aid in weight loss.

**Ingredients:**

**Jeera (cumin seeds):** Harness the power of cumin seeds, known for their potential digestive benefits and distinct flavour, servs as the primary ingredient in the Jeera Detox Water.

**Method:**

To create the "Jeera Detox Water," follow these simple steps:

**Soak Cumin Seeds:** Take 1-2 teaspoons of cumin seeds and soak them in a glass of water. Allow the cumin seeds to infuse into the water by soaking overnight.

**Strain and Drink:** In the morning, strain the water to remove the cumin seeds. Drink the infused jeera water on an empty stomach for maximum benefits.

**Benefits:**

**Effortless Detoxification:** Jeera Detox Water offers a straightforward and uncomplicated method for detoxifying your body, requiring minimal time and effort in its preparation.

**Digestive Support:** Cumin seeds are known for their potential digestive benefits, including aiding digestion and reducing bloating, contributing to a healthier gut.

**Weight Loss Aid:** Incorporating jeera water into your routine offers support in weight loss efforts. The combination of cumin's properties and the hydration aspect of the water can contribute to a balanced approach to weight management.

**Antioxidant Properties:** Cumin seeds contain antioxidants that may help combat oxidative stress in the body, promoting overall health.

**Hydration Boost:** Jeera Detox Water serves as a hydrating beverage, supporting optimal fluid balance and helping you stay refreshed throughout the day.

Enjoy the benefits of Jeera Detox Water as a delightful addition to your daily routine.

*Cheers to simplicity and well-being!*

# 20

## Tomato Detox Drink

Elevate your detox journey with the invigorating "Tomato Detox Drink," a refreshing blend of natural tomato juice and the zesty essence of lemon. This low-calorie concoction not only tantalizes your taste buds but also brings a burst of diuretic properties from lemon, potentially aiding in weight loss. Served on ice, this revitalizjking drink offers a delightful way to stay hydrated and refreshed while enjoying the benefits of vitamin C.

**Ingredients:**

**Natural, Pre-made Tomato Juice (150 ml):** Embrace the rich flavour and nutritional benefits of natural tomato juice, serving as the base for this detox drink.

**Lemon Juice (25 ml):** Introduce the citrusy freshness of lemon juice, which not only enhances the flavour but also contributes diuretic properties and a dose of vitamin C.

**Mineral Water:** Complete the blend with mineral water, which provides a crisp and hydrating element to the detox drink.

**Method of Preparation:**

Follow these simple steps while preparing the "Tomato Detox Drink,":

**Mix the Ingredients in a Cup:** Combine 150 ml of natural, pre-made tomato juice with 25 ml of lemon juice in a cup.

**Add Mineral Water:** Pour mineral water into the cup, adjusting the quantity according to your preference for dilution.

**Drink on Ice:** Serve the detox drink over ice, enhancing the refreshing quality and ensuring a cool and invigorating experience.

**Storage:** As this drink contains vitamin C, it can be stored in a sealed container and refrigerated for up to six hours, allowing you to enjoy its benefits throughout the day.

**Benefits:**

**Diuretic Properties of Lemon:** Lemon's diuretic properties help in weight loss by promoting the elimination of excess fluids from the body.

**Low-Calorie Refreshment:** With only about 30 calories per cup, this detox drink provides a flavourful and low-calorie alternative for those seeking a refreshing beverage.

**Vitamin C Boost:** The inclusion of lemon juice contributes vitamin C to the drink, offering immune-boosting benefits and enhancing overall well-being.

Indulge in the "Tomato Detox Drink," relish its unique blend of flavours and benefit from its hydrating and refreshing qualities. Whether enjoyed over ice or stored for later, let this delightful concoction be a part of your wellness routine.

*Cheers to healthful sipping!*

# 21

# Water, Cashew and Cinnamon Juice Detox

Embark on a journey of flavour and wellness with the "Water, Cashew, and Cinnamon Juice Detox," a harmonious blend of hydrating watermelon, zesty lemon, the tropical essence of coconut water, the warmth of cinnamon, and the richness of cashews. Beyond its delicious taste, this detox juice is designed to elevate your metabolism and support fat-burning, making it a delightful addition to your health and wellness routine.

**Ingredients:**

**Watermelon (1 medium slice):** Embrace the hydrating and refreshing qualities of watermelon, forming the juicy base for this detox juice.

**Lemon Juice (Juice of 1 lemon):** Introduce a burst of citrusy freshness with lemon juice, which enhances the overall flavour profile and contributes potential digestive benefits.

**Coconut Water (150 ml):** Infuse the juice with the tropical goodness of coconut water, providing hydration and a subtle sweetness.

**Cinnamon (1 teaspoon):** Add warmth and thermogenic properties with cinnamon, potentially boosting metabolism and promoting fat burning.

**Cashews (1 small handful):** Incorporate the creamy richness of cashews, adding a satisfying texture and potential nutritional benefits.

**Method of preparation:**

To prepare the "Water, Cashew, and Cinnamon Juice Detox," follow these simple steps:

**Blend Ingredients:** In a blender, mix the medium slice of watermelon, lemon juice, coconut water, cinnamon, and a handful of cashews. Blend until all the ingredients are well combined.

**Strain and Drink:** Strain the blended mixture to achieve a smooth consistency. Drink the juice, preferably without sweetener, allowing the natural flavours to shine.

**Storage:** This juice can be stored in a well-sealed container in refrigerator for up to six hours, offering a convenient and refreshing option throughout the day.

**Benefits:**

**Metabolism Boost with Cinnamon:** Cinnamon's thermogenic actions enhance metabolism, potentially increase fat burning and support weight management.

**Hydration and Refreshment:** Watermelon and coconut water contribute to the hydrating and refreshing qualities of the juice, making it a delightful choice for staying hydrated.

**Nutrient-Rich Cashews:** Cashews bring a handful of creamy richness to the mix, offering potential nutritional benefits and adding a satisfying texture.

**Calorie-Conscious Option:** With approximately 83 calories per 250 mL serving, this detox juice provides a flavourful and calorie-conscious alternative for those seeking a healthful beverage.

Indulge in the "Water, Cashew, and Cinnamon Juice Detox," relish its unique blend of flavours and embrace the potential benefits it brings to your wellness journey.

*Sip, enjoy, and toast to healthful living!*

# 22

# Hibiscus Juice with Strawberries Detox

Revitalize your senses and indulge in the vibrant hues of the "Hibiscus Juice with Strawberries Detox," a refreshing elixir that combines the floral notes of hibiscus tea with the sweet and tangy essence of strawberries. Beyond its delightful taste, this detox juice harnesses the diuretic properties of hibiscus, potentially aiding in fluid excretion and contributing to weight loss. With approximately 21 calories per 250 mL serving, it stands as a flavourful and calorie-conscious option for those embracing a healthful beverage.

**Ingredients:**

**Hibiscus Tea (1 cup):** Infuse the detox with the rich and floral notes of hibiscus tea, providing a vibrant base for the beverage.

**Strawberries (5 numbers):** Introduce the luscious sweetness and vibrant colour of strawberries, elevating the overall flavour profile and contributing potential nutritional benefits.

**Method of Preparation:**

In the preparation of "Hibiscus Juice with Strawberries Detox," follow these simple steps:

**Prepare Strawberries:** Wash the strawberries, remove the leaves, and dice them into smaller pieces.

**Blend Ingredients:** In a blender, combine the diced strawberries and hibiscus tea. Blend until the ingredients are well combined, creating a smooth and vibrant mixture.

**Pour and Drink:** Pour the blended juice into a cup and enjoy it, preferably without sweetener, allowing the natural flavours to shine.

**Storage:** This juice can be stored in a well-sealed container in the refrigerator for up to six hours, offering a convenient and refreshing option throughout the day.

**Benefits:**

**Diuretic Properties of Hibiscus:** Hibiscus tea's diuretic properties aid in the excretion of body fluids, potentially supporting weight loss and fluid balance.

**Strawberries' Sweet and Tangy Essence:** Strawberries contribute a sweet and tangy flavour to the detox, enhancing the overall taste and providing potential nutritional benefits.

**Calorie-Conscious Option:** With approximately 21 calories per 250 mL serving, this detox juice offers a flavourful and calorie-conscious alternative for those mindful of their calorie intake.

Indulge in the "Hibiscus Juice with Strawberries Detox," savour the delightful combination of flavours and embrace the potential benefits it brings to your wellness routine.

*Sip, enjoy, and toast to vibrant living!*

# 23

# Watermelon and Ginger Juice Detox

Embark on a journey of hydration and well-being with the "Watermelon and Ginger Juice Detox," a refreshing elixir that combines the hydrating essence of watermelon, the fibre-rich goodness of flaxseeds, and the zesty warmth of fresh ginger. Beyond its delicious taste, this detox juice offers potential benefits for bloating and appetite control, making it a flavourful and healthful addition to your wellness routine. With approximately 130 calories per 250 mL serving, it stands as a nourishing choice for those seeking a satisfying beverage.

**Ingredients:**

**Watermelon (2 slices, seedless):** Embrace the juicy and hydrating qualities of seedless watermelon, serving as the base for this detox juice.

**Flaxseeds (1 teaspoon, ground):** Introduce the fibre-rich goodness of ground flaxseeds, contributing to potential benefits for bloating and appetite control.

**Ginger (1 teaspoon, fresh, grated):** Add a zesty and warming touch to the juice with fresh, grated ginger, providing not only flavour but also potential digestive benefits.

**Method of preparation:**

Follow these simple steps in the preparation of "Watermelon and Ginger Juice Detox".

**Blend the Ingredients:** In a blender, combine the two slices of seedless watermelon, ground flaxseeds (1 teaspoon), and fresh, grated ginger (1 teaspoon). Blend until all the ingredients are well combined.

**Strain and Drink:** Strain the blended mixture to achieve a smooth consistency. Drink the juice without sweetening, allowing the natural flavours to shine.

**Storage:** This detox drink can be stored in a well-sealed container in refrigerator for up to six hours, offering a convenient and refreshing option throughout the day.

**Benefits:**

**Hydrating Watermelon:** Watermelon's high water content contributes to hydration, making it a refreshing choice and potentially aiding in appetite control.

**Fibre-Rich Flaxseeds:** Ground flaxseeds bring fibre to the mix, potentially supporting digestive health, bloating reduction, and appetite control.

**Zesty Digestive Boost with Ginger:** Fresh, grated ginger adds a zesty and warming element to the juice, providing potential digestive benefits and enhancing overall well-being.

**Calorie-Conscious Option:** With approximately 130 calories per 250 mL serving, this detox juice offers a satisfying and calorie-conscious alternative for those mindful of their calorie intake.

Indulge in the "Watermelon and Ginger Juice Detox," relish its unique blend of flavours and embrace the potential benefits it brings to your wellness journey.

*Sip, enjoy, and toast to healthful living!*

# 24

## Cabbage, Beet and Ginger Juice Detox

Embark on a journey of detoxification and vitality with the "Cabbage, Beet, and Ginger Juice Detox," a nutrient-rich elixir that combines the fluid-eliminating properties of cucumber and cabbage, the vibrant earthiness of beet and the metabolism-boosting warmth of fresh, grated ginger. Beyond its vibrant flavour, this detox juice aids in fat-burning and weight loss, offering a satisfying and healthful option with approximately 100 calories per 250 mL serving.

**Ingredients:**

**Cabbage Leaves (2 numbers):** Embrace the detoxifying properties of cabbage leaves, contributing to the elimination of excess fluid in the body.

**Mint Leaves (1 tablespoon, fresh):** Introduce a refreshing touch with fresh mint leaves, enhances the overall flavour profile of the juice.

**Beet (1 small):** Add a vibrant hue and nutrient-rich beet to the mix, contributing potential benefits for detoxification.

**Cucumber (1/2, with peel):** Incorporate the hydrating and fluid-eliminating properties of cucumber, which enhances the overall freshness of the juice.

**Ginger (1 teaspoon, fresh, grated):** Infuse the juice with the warming essence of fresh, grated ginger, which potentially accelerates metabolism and aids in fat-burning.

**Water (1 cup):** Provides the base for the juice with a cup of water, also ensures a smooth and hydrating consistency.

**Methods of Preparation:**

To prepare the "Cabbage, Beet, and Ginger Juice Detox," follow these simple steps:

**Prepare Ingredients:** Wash the cabbage leaves, mint leaves, beet, and cucumber thoroughly. Peel the beet and cut both the beet and cucumber into cubes.

**Blend Ingredients:** In a blender, combine the cubed beet and cucumber with the cabbage leaves, fresh mint leaves, fresh, grated ginger, and water. Blend for approximately three minutes or until all the ingredients are well mixed.

**Strain and Drink:** Strain the blended mixture to achieve a smooth consistency. Drink the juice, preferably without sweetener, allowing the natural flavours to shine.

**Storage:** This juice can be stored in an air tight container in the refrigerator for up to six hours, providing a convenient and refreshing option throughout the day.

**Benefits:**

**Fluid Elimination with Cucumber and Cabbage:** Cucumber and cabbage contribute in eliminating excess fluid in the body, potentially aiding in detoxification.

**Metabolism Boost with Ginger:** Fresh, grated ginger adds a warming element to the juice, potentially accelerating metabolism and supporting fat-burning.

**Nutrient-Rich Beet:** Beet brings a vibrant colour and nutrient-rich profile to the juice, offering potential detoxification benefits.

**Calorie-Conscious Option:** With approximately 100 calories per 250 mL serving, this detox juice stands as a satisfying and calorie-conscious alternative for those mindful of their calorie intake.

Indulge in the "Cabbage, Beet, and Ginger Juice Detox," savouring its unique combination of flavours and embracing the potential benefits it brings to your wellness journey.

*Sip, enjoy, and toast to vibrant living!*

# 25

## Strawberry Spinach Detox Drink

Elevate your wellness journey with the invigorating "Strawberry Spinach Detox Drink," a vibrant elixir that blends the sweet essence of strawberries with the nutrient-rich goodness of spinach. Packed with antioxidants and essential vitamins, this refreshing beverage not only tantalizes your taste buds but also offers potential benefits for detoxification and overall well-being. Embrace the natural goodness of these ingredients as you sip your way to a healthier, revitalized life.

**Ingredients:**

**Strawberries (1 cup, hulled):** Introduce the sweet and juicy flavour of strawberries, rich in vitamin C and antioxidants, contributing to the drink's refreshing taste and potential health benefits.

**Spinach (1 cup, fresh):** Harness the nutrient power of fresh spinach, packed with vitamins, minerals, and antioxidants, providing a green boost to your detox drink.

**Lemon (1, juiced):** Add a zesty kick with freshly squeezed lemon juice, enhancing the overall flavour and contributing potential detoxifying properties.

**Cucumber (1/2, sliced):** Incorporate the hydrating and cleansing properties of cucumber, contributing to the drink's refreshing quality.

**Mint Leaves (a handful, fresh):** Introduce a burst of freshness with fresh mint leaves, enhancing the overall aroma and flavour of the detox drink.

**Water (2 cups):** Serve as the hydrating base, ensuring a smooth and well-balanced consistency.

**Method of Preparation:**

We should follow these simple steps while preparing the "Strawberry Spinach Detox Drink":

**Prepare Ingredients:** Hull the strawberries, slice the cucumber, and squeeze the lemon.

**Blend Ingredients:** In a blender, combine the hulled strawberries, fresh spinach, sliced cucumber, freshly squeezed lemon juice, fresh mint leaves, and water. Blend until all the ingredients are well combined and the mixture reaches a smooth consistency.

**Strain (Optional):** If desired, strain the blended mixture to achieve a smoother texture.

**Serve and Enjoy:** Pour the detox drink into glasses and savour the refreshing goodness. Serve over ice if preferred.

**Benefits:**

**Antioxidant Power:** Strawberries and spinach are rich in antioxidants, which help combat oxidative stress and support overall health.

**Hydration and Cleansing:** Cucumbers and lemons contribute to hydration and cleansing, aiding in detoxification and promoting a refreshed feeling.

**Nutrient Boost:** Spinach brings essential vitamins and minerals to the mix, enhancing the nutritional profile of the detox drink.

**Digestive Support:** Mint leaves add a delightful touch and contribute to digestive comfort, enhancing the overall wellness experience.

Embrace the rejuvenating qualities of the "Strawberry Spinach Detox Drink," allowing its vibrant flavours and potential health benefits to revitalize your senses.

*Sip, enjoy, and toast to a healthier life!*

# 26

# Detoxifying Carrot-Banana Bliss Smoothie

Elevate your daily refreshment with the "Detoxifying Carrot-Banana Bliss Smoothie," a plant-powered elixir designed to delight your taste buds while supporting your body's natural detoxification process. This vegan concoction seamlessly blends the wholesome sweetness of ripe bananas with the earthy goodness of freshly grated carrots, creating a smoothie that not only satisfies cravings but also contributes to your overall well-being. With detoxifying ingredients like chia seeds and a hint of optional natural sweetener, this smoothie is a delicious and healthful addition to your routine.

**Ingredients:**

**Ripe Bananas (two, peeled and sliced):** Infuse natural sweetness and creaminess into the smoothie, providing a delightful base.

**Carrots (one cup, grated):** Introduce the detoxifying power of carrots, rich in antioxidants and vitamins that support the body's cleansing processes.

**Almond Milk (one cup):** Create a dairy-free and luscious base, ensuring a smooth and enjoyable texture.

**Chia Seeds (1 tablespoon):** Enhance the detox benefits with chia seeds, known for their fibre content and ability to support digestive health.

**Maple Syrup or Agave Nectar (1-2 tablespoons, optional):** Optionally sweeten the smoothie with a natural touch, allowing you to tailor the sweetness according to your preference.

**Ice Cubes (optional):** Boost the refreshing quality of the smoothie by adding ice cubes, which create a cool and revitalizing treat.

**Method of preparation:**

To prepare the "Detoxifying Carrot-Banana Bliss Smoothie," follow these steps:

**Prepare Ingredients:** Peel and slice the ripe bananas, grate carrots, and gather all other ingredients.

**Blend Ingredients:** In a blender, combine sliced bananas, grated carrots, almond milk, chia seeds, and optional sweetener. Blend until achieving a smooth and creamy consistency.

**Adjust Consistency:** For an added refreshing element, include ice cubes if needed. Blend again until the ice is fully incorporated.

**Serve and Enjoy:** Pour the detoxifying smoothie into glasses, garnish with a carrot slice or banana wheel if desired, and relish the blissful fusion of flavours.

**Benefits:**

**Antioxidant-Rich Carrots:** Grated carrots provide antioxidants that aid in detoxification, supporting the body's natural cleansing processes.

**Fibre-Packed Chia Seeds:** Chia seeds contribute to the detoxifying process by providing ample fibre, and promoting healthy digestion.

**Hydrating Almond Milk:** The almond milk base ensures hydration, essential for flushing toxins from the body.

**Vegan and Dairy-Free Delight:** Suitable for vegans, this smoothie provides a dairy-free alternative for those seeking plant-based options.

**Customizable Sweetness:** The optional addition of natural sweeteners like maple syrup or agave nectar allows you to customize the sweetness to your liking.

Embrace the revitalizing qualities of the "Detoxifying Carrot-Banana Bliss Smoothie," a delicious fusion of detoxifying ingredients crafted to enhance your well-being.

*Sip, savour, and toast to a healthier, refreshed life!*

# 27

## Autumn Harvest Bliss Smoothie

Embark on a journey through the crisp essence of fall with the "Autumn Harvest Bliss Smoothie." This delightful concoction captures the warm and comforting flavours of a classic pumpkin pie, blending them into a nourishing and invigorating smoothie. Immerse yourself in the richness of seasonal ingredients, welcoming the spirit of autumn with every sip. This smoothie is not just a beverage; it's a celebration of the harvest season, offering a blissful fusion of taste and nutrition.

**Ingredients:**

**Pumpkin Puree (1/2 cup):** Infuse the smoothie with the creamy richness of pumpkin, a quintessential fall ingredient that brings both flavour and nutrition.

**Banana (one, ripe):** Adds natural sweetness and creaminess to the blend, complements pumpkin and provides essential vitamins.

**Almond Milk (one cup):** Create a luscious and dairy-free base, ensuring a smooth and velvety texture to the smoothie.

**Maple Syrup (1-2 tablespoons, to taste):** Enhance the autumn sweetness with pure maple syrup, which offers a natural and indulgent touch.

**Ground Cinnamon (1/2 teaspoon):** Introduce the warm and comforting spice of cinnamon, reminiscent of traditional pumpkin pie seasoning.

**Vanilla Extract (1/2 teaspoon):** Elevate the flavour profile with a hint of vanilla extract, adding a subtle sweetness and aromatic essence.

**Ice Cubes (optional):** Enhance the refreshing quality of the smoothie by adding ice cubes, creating a cool and invigorating treat.

**Method of Preparation:**

To create the "Autumn Harvest Bliss Smoothie," follow these simple steps:

**Prepare Ingredients:** Gather the pumpkin puree, ripe banana, almond milk, maple syrup, ground cinnamon, vanilla extract, and optional ice cubes.

**Blend Ingredients:** In a blender, combine the pumpkin puree, ripe banana, almond milk, maple syrup, ground cinnamon, and vanilla extract. Blend until the mixture reaches a smooth and velvety consistency.

**Adjust Sweetness:** Taste the smoothie and adjust the sweetness according to your preference by adding more maple syrup if desired.

**Add Ice Cubes (Optional):** For a cooler and more refreshing experience, include ice cubes and blend again until well incorporated.

**Serve and Enjoy:** Pour the Autumn Harvest Bliss Smoothie into glasses, savour the rich flavours, and let the essence of fall embrace your senses.

**Benefits:**

**Nutrient-Rich Pumpkin:** Canned pumpkin puree is a powerhouse of nutrients, including vitamins A and C, contributing to immune health and skin vitality.

**Potassium from Banana:** The ripe banana adds potassium, supporting heart health and maintaining proper fluid balance in the body.

**Dairy-Free Indulgence:** Almond milk provides a dairy-free alternative, making this smoothie suitable for those with lactose intolerance or following a vegan lifestyle.

**Natural Sweetening with Maple Syrup:** Pure maple syrup serves as a natural sweetener, offering a deliciously indulgent touch without refined sugars.

**Warm and Comforting Spices:** Ground cinnamon and vanilla extract bring a cosy and comforting element to the smoothie, enhancing the overall sensory experience.

Celebrate the flavours of autumn with the "Autumn Harvest Bliss Smoothie," a wholesome and delicious blend that captures the essence of the season.

*Sip, savour, and immerse yourself in the blissful embrace of fall.*

# 28

# Eternal Green Vitality Elixir

Revitalize your body and refresh your senses with the "Eternal Green Vitality Elixir", a vibrant concoction that merges the nutrient-packed goodness of spinach with the creamy richness of avocado. This detox drink goes beyond the ordinary, offering a symphony of flavours that not only cleanse but also nourish our body and mind. Dive into the invigorating fusion of green vitality as each sip brings you closer to a rejuvenated and energized version of yourself.

**Ingredients:**

**Fresh Spinach (2 cups):** Harness the detoxifying power of fresh spinach, loaded with antioxidants and essential nutrients that support overall health.

**Avocado (1, ripe):** Introduce creamy texture and healthy fats with ripe avocado, contributing to a smooth and satisfying consistency.

**Cucumber (1/2, sliced):** Infuse hydration and a crisp element with cucumber, promoting detoxification and refreshing the palate.

**Lemon (1, juiced):** Add a burst of citrusy brightness with freshly squeezed lemon juice, enhancing the overall flavour profile and offering detox benefits.

**Mint Leaves (a handful):** Elevate the freshness with mint leaves, known for their digestive properties and delightful aroma.

**Ginger (1/2 inch, grated):** Incorporate the zing of ginger, renowned for its anti-inflammatory properties and potential detoxifying effects.

**Water two cups):** Serve as the hydrating base, ensuring a smooth and well-balanced consistency for the detox elixir.

**Method of preparation:**

To prepare the "Eternal Green Vitality Elixir," follow these straightforward steps:

**Prepare Ingredients:** Wash and gather the fresh spinach, ripe avocado, cucumber, lemon, mint leaves, and ginger.

**Blend Ingredients:** In a blender, combine the fresh spinach, peeled and pitted avocado, sliced cucumber, freshly squeezed lemon juice, mint leaves, grated ginger, and water. Blend until achieving a smooth and velvety consistency.

**Adjust Consistency:** If needed, add more water to reach your preferred thickness, and blend again until well incorporated.

**Serve and Enjoy:** Pour the Eternal Green Vitality Elixir into glasses, perhaps over ice, for an extra refreshing touch. Garnish with a sprig of mint or cucumber slice, and relish the revitalizing flavours.

**Benefits:**

**Antioxidant Boost from Spinach:** Fresh spinach provides a robust dose of antioxidants, supporting the body's defence against oxidative stress.

**Healthy Fats and Creaminess from Avocado:** Ripe avocado contributes heart-healthy monounsaturated fats, adding creaminess and satiety to the elixir.

**Hydration and Detox from Cucumber:** Cucumber's high water content aids in hydration, while its natural diuretic properties support detoxification.

**Citrus Detox with Lemon:** Lemon juice enhances the detoxifying effect with its citrusy brightness and potential alkalizing properties.

**Digestive Comfort from Mint and Ginger:** Mint leaves and grated ginger introduce digestive benefits, promoting comfort and aiding in the detox process.

**Nutrient-Rich Refreshment:** The combination of these ingredients results in a nutrient-rich elixir, offering a delicious and healthful way to revitalize your body.

Embark on a journey of rejuvenation with the " Eternal Green Vitality Elixir," a green elixir that not only detoxifies but also delights your senses.

*Sip, savour, and embrace the vitality it brings to your well-being.*

# 29

## Zesty Citrus Pineapple Cleanse

Embark on a journey of rejuvenation with the "Zesty Citrus Pineapple Cleanse," a vibrant detox drink that harmoniously blends the tropical sweetness of pineapple with the refreshing zest of orange. This invigorating concoction not only tantalizes your taste buds but also revitalizes your body, offering a burst of citrusy delight with each sip. Elevate your wellness routine as you indulge in this clean and cleansing elixir, embracing the tropical symphony of flavours that promise a refreshing escape.

**Ingredients:**

- **Fresh Pineapple (1 cup, diced):** Infuse tropical sweetness with fresh pineapple, rich in vitamins and enzymes that support digestion.
- **Oranges (two, peeled and segmented):** Introduce a burst of citrusy goodness with oranges, packed with vitamin C and antioxidants for immune support.
- **Cucumber (1/2, sliced):** Enhance hydration and add a crisp element with cucumber, known for its refreshing properties.
- **Mint Leaves (a handful):** Elevate freshness with mint leaves, offering a soothing aroma and potential digestive benefits.
- **Ginger (1/2 inch, grated):** Incorporate the zing of ginger, celebrated for its anti-inflammatory properties and digestive support.

**Water (two cups):** Serve as the hydrating base, ensuring a well-balanced and smooth consistency for the detox drink.

**Method of preparation:**

To prepare the "Zesty Citrus Pineapple Cleanse," follow these simple steps:

**Prepare Ingredients:** Wash and dice fresh pineapple, peel and segment oranges, slice cucumber, add mint leaves, and grated ginger.

**Blend Ingredients:** In a blender, combine the fresh pineapple, orange segments, cucumber slices, mint leaves, grated ginger, and water. Blend until achieving a smooth and refreshing consistency.

**Strain (Optional):** If a smoother texture is preferred, strain the mixture to remove the pulp. Otherwise, enjoy the drink with its natural fibre content.

**Serve and Garnish:** Pour the Zesty Citrus Pineapple Cleanse into glasses, perhaps over ice for added refreshment. Garnish with a mint sprig or a slice of pineapple for an extra touch of tropical allure.

**Benefits:**

**Vitamin C Boost:** Oranges and pineapple are rich in vitamin C, promoting immune health and providing antioxidant support.

**Hydration Support:** Cucumber's high water content contributes to hydration, supporting overall well-being.

**Digestive Comfort:** The combination of mint leaves and ginger may offer digestive benefits, promoting comfort and aiding in digestion.

**Antioxidant Richness:** Pineapple and oranges bring a wealth of antioxidants, assisting the body in combating oxidative stress.

**Refreshing Detox:** The natural flavours and properties of the ingredients create a refreshing detox drink, perfect for cleansing and revitalizing the body.

Sip into a tropical sanctuary of wellness with the "Zesty Citrus Pineapple Cleanse," a delightful concoction that promises both refreshment and rejuvenation.

Embrace the vibrant fusion of flavours and bask in the uplifting benefits of this citrus-infused elixir.

# 30

## Tropical Cauliflower Revitalizer Smoothie

Embark on a journey of unexpected yet delightful flavours with the "Tropical Cauliflower Revitalizer Smoothie," a unique and nutritious blend that seamlessly blends the tropical essence of fruits with the wholesome goodness of cauliflower. This unconventional smoothie invites you to experience the harmonious fusion of sweet and savoury notes, promising a refreshing and revitalizing sip that challenges traditional expectations. Elevate your wellness routine with this innovative concoction, celebrating the vibrant synergy of tropical indulgence and cruciferous nourishment.

**Ingredients:**

**Frozen Pineapple Chunks (one cup):** Infuse tropical sweetness and vitamins into the smoothie, creating a luscious base.

**Mango (1/2, diced):** Introduce another layer of tropical flavour with ripe mango, adding natural sweetness and fibre.

**Cauliflower Florets (1/2 cup):** Incorporate the unexpected yet nutritious element of cauliflower, providing a creamy texture and an array of health benefits.

**Coconut Milk (one cup):** Enhance the tropical profile and creaminess with coconut milk, offering a rich and indulgent base.

**Banana (1, ripe):** Add natural sweetness and creaminess to the smoothie, contributing potassium and essential vitamins.

**Chia Seeds (1 tablespoon):** Boost the nutritional content with chia seeds, delivering omega-3 fatty acids, fibre, and a subtle crunch.

**Lime Juice (1 tablespoon):** Introduce a zesty and citrusy twist with lime juice, elevating the overall flavour profile.

**Method:**

To prepare the "Tropical Cauliflower Revitalizer Smoothie," follow these straightforward steps:

**Prepare Ingredients:** Gather frozen pineapple chunks, diced mango, cauliflower florets, coconut milk, a ripe banana, chia seeds, and lime juice.

**Blending Process:** In a blender, combine the frozen pineapple chunks, diced mango, cauliflower florets, coconut milk, ripe banana, chia seeds, and lime juice.

Blend Until Smooth: Blend the ingredients until achieving a smooth and velvety consistency, ensuring the cauliflower is fully incorporated.

Adjust Consistency (Optional): If a thicker or thinner consistency is desired, adjust by adding more coconut milk or water and blend again.

**Serve and Enjoy:** Pour the Tropical Cauliflower Revitalizer Smoothie into glasses, perhaps over ice for an extra refreshing touch. Garnish with a pineapple slice or a sprinkle of chia seeds for visual appeal.

**Benefits:**

**Cruciferous Goodness of Cauliflower:** Cauliflower contributes essential nutrients, including vitamins C and K, and provide antioxidant and anti-inflammatory benefits.

**Tropical Vitamin Boost:** Pineapple and mango bring a wealth of vitamins, particularly vitamin C, supporting immune health and overall well-being.

**Creamy Coconut Nutrients:** Coconut milk provides a creamy base rich in healthy fats, contributing to satiety and providing sustained energy.

**Hydration from Fruits:** The natural water content in pineapple, mango, and banana aids in hydration, promoting optimal bodily functions.

**Omega-3 and Fibre from Chia Seeds:** Chia seeds offer omega-3 fatty acids and fibre, supporting heart health and digestive well-being.

**Refreshing Zest with Lime:** Lime juice adds a refreshing and citrusy element, enhancing the overall taste experience.

Embrace the unexpected and savour the nourishing fusion of flavours in the "Tropical Cauliflower Revitalizer Smoothie," a testament to the innovative world of smoothie creations. Indulge in this unique blend that not only surprises your palate but also nourishes your body with a spectrum of healthful benefits.

# 31

# Verde Vitality Kale and Apple Detox Blend

Embark on a journey of vibrant wellness with the "Verde Vitality Kale & Apple Detox Blend," a refreshing elixir that combines the wholesome richness of kale with the crisp sweetness of apples. This invigorating blend is crafted to elevate your detox experience, providing a symphony of flavours that not only tantalize your taste buds but also nourish your body. Immerse yourself in the verdant embrace of this detox blend, where kale's nutritional prowess meets the delightful essence of fresh apples for a rejuvenating sip.

**Ingredients:**

**Fresh Kale Leaves (two cups, destemmed):** Harness the nutritional powerhouse of kale, rich in vitamins, minerals, and antioxidants, promoting overall well-being.

**Sweet Apples (two, cored and sliced):** Introduce natural sweetness and a hint of tartness with fresh apples, providing vitamins and fibre for a delightful taste.

**Cucumber (1/2, sliced):** Enhance hydration and add a crisp element with cucumber, contributing to the detoxifying properties of the blend.

**Lemon Juice (1 tablespoon):** Infuse a zesty and citrusy brightness with freshly squeezed lemon juice, enhancing the overall flavour profile.

**Ginger (1/2 inch, grated):** Incorporate the invigorating warmth of ginger, known for its anti-inflammatory and digestive benefits.

**Chia Seeds (one tablespoon):** Boost the nutritional content with chia seeds, which offer omega-3 fatty acids, fibre, and a subtle crunch.

**Coconut Water (one cup):** Provide a hydrating base with coconut water, adding a tropical touch and replenishing electrolytes.

**Method:**

To prepare the "Verde Vitality Kale & Apple Detox Blend," follow these simple steps:

**Prepare Ingredients:** De-stem the kale leaves, core and slice apples, slice cucumber, grate ginger, and gather lemon juice, chia seeds, and coconut water.

**Blending Process:** In a blender, combine the destemmed kale leaves, sliced apples, cucumber slices, freshly grated ginger, lemon juice, chia seeds, and coconut water.

**Blend Until Smooth:** Blend the ingredients until achieving a smooth and velvety consistency, ensuring the kale is fully incorporated.

**Adjust Consistency (Optional):** If a thicker or thinner consistency is desired, adjust by adding more coconut water or water and blend again.

**Serve and Enjoy:** Pour the Verde Vitality Kale & Apple Detox Blend into glasses, perhaps over ice, for an extra refreshing touch. Garnish with a kale leaf or apple slice for an elegant presentation.

**Benefits:**

**Kale's Nutrient Density:** Kale provides a concentrated source of vitamins A, C, and K, along with minerals and antioxidants, supporting immune health and overall vitality.

**Apple's Natural Sweetness:** Apples bring natural sweetness and dietary fibre, aiding digestion and providing essential vitamins and minerals.

**Hydration and Electrolytes:** Coconut water serves as a hydrating base, replenishing electrolytes and contributing to overall hydration.

**Detoxifying Properties:** Cucumber's high-water content and kale's detoxifying properties support the body's natural detox processes.

**Anti-Inflammatory Ginger:** Ginger adds an anti-inflammatory component, potentially aiding digestion and providing a warming sensation.

**Omega-3 and Fibre from Chia Seeds:** Chia seeds offer omega-3 fatty acids and fibre, promoting heart health and digestive well-being.

Savour the invigorating embrace of healthful ingredients in the "Verde Vitality Kale & Apple Detox Blend," a fusion of greens and sweetness designed to revitalize your body and delight your palate.

Embrace the verdant essence of this detox elixir, celebrating the nourishing synergy it brings to your wellness routine.

# 32

# Cruciferous Cleanse Fusion

Embark on a journey of detoxification and revitalization with the "Cruciferous Cleanse Fusion," a vibrant smoothie that harmoniously blends the robust flavours of broccoli, the earthy richness of beets, and the nutrient-packed freshness of spinach. This unique fusion not only excites your taste buds but also nourishes your body with a symphony of vitamins, minerals, and antioxidants. Elevate your well-being with this wholesome concoction, where the cruciferous power of broccoli meets the vibrant hues of beets and the leafy goodness of spinach for a refreshing cleanse.

**Ingredients:**

**Fresh Broccoli Florets (one cup):** Harness the detoxifying properties and nutritional richness of broccoli, packed with vitamins C and K, fibre, and antioxidants.

**Beets (1 medium-sized, peeled and diced):** Introduce a vibrant burst of colour and earthy sweetness with beets, providing essential nutrients like folate and manganese.

**Spinach Leaves (2 cups):** Add a dose of leafy goodness with fresh spinach, contributing vitamins A, C, and K, as well as iron and folate.

**Banana (one, ripe):** Infuse natural sweetness and creaminess with a ripe banana, offering potassium, vitamins, and energy.

**Greek Yogurt (1/2 cup):** Provide a creamy texture and additional nutrients with Greek yoghurt, supplying probiotics for gut health.

**Chia Seeds (one tablespoon):** Boost the nutritional content with chia seeds, delivering omega-3 fatty acids, fibre, and a subtle crunch.

**Almond Milk (one cup):** Create a smooth and dairy-free base with almond milk, offering a nutty flavour and essential nutrients.

**Method of preparation:**

To prepare the "Cruciferous Cleanse Fusion," follow these simple steps:

**Preparation of Ingredients:** Cut broccoli into florets, peel and dice the beet, measure spinach leaves, peel the ripe banana, and gather Greek yoghurt, chia seeds, and almond milk.

**Blending Process:** In a blender, combine the broccoli florets, diced beet, spinach leaves, ripe banana, Greek yoghurt, chia seeds, and almond milk.

**Blend Until Smooth:** Blend the ingredients until achieving a smooth and velvety consistency, ensuring the cruciferous components are fully incorporated.

**Adjust Consistency (Optional):** If a thicker or thinner consistency is needed, adjust by adding more almond milk or water and blend again.

**Serve and Enjoy:** Pour the Cruciferous Cleanse Fusion into glasses, perhaps over ice for an extra refreshing touch. Garnish with a beet slice or a sprinkle of chia seeds for visual appeal.

**Benefits:**

**Detoxifying Cruciferous Power:** Broccoli's compounds support the body's natural detoxification processes, aiding in overall cleansing.

**Vibrant Beet Nutrients:** Beets provide a rich source of antioxidants, vitamins, and minerals, potentially supporting heart health and energy.

**Leafy Goodness from Spinach:** Spinach contributes to the smoothie's nutrient profile with vitamins, iron, and folate, promoting overall well-being.

**Natural Sweetness and Potassium:** The ripe banana adds natural sweetness and potassium, supporting muscle function and heart health.

**Probiotics from Greek Yoghurt:** Greek yoghurt introduces probiotics, promoting a healthy gut microbiome and aiding digestion.

**Omega-3 and Fibre from Chia Seeds:** Chia seeds offer omega-3 fatty acids and fibre, supporting heart health and digestive well-being.

**Dairy-Free Nutrients:** Almond milk provides a dairy-free base with essential nutrients like vitamin E and calcium.

Immerse yourself in the vibrant hues and nourishing benefits of the "Cruciferous Cleanse Fusion," a smoothie designed to cleanse and revitalize your body with the wholesome goodness of cruciferous vegetables, beets, and spinach. Celebrate the fusion of flavours and healthful properties as you embrace this refreshing addition to your wellness routine.

# 33

# Mango Green Revitalizer Blend

Energize your senses and embrace a burst of tropical goodness with the "Mango Green Revitalizer Blend," a delightful smoothie that merges the luscious sweetness of mangoes with the vibrant freshness of spinach. This invigorating blend is a celebration of flavours and nourishment, offering a refreshing escape to a tropical paradise while providing your body with a wealth of essential vitamins and minerals. Immerse yourself in the revitalizing fusion of mango and spinach, crafted to elevate your well-being and awaken your taste buds.

**Ingredients:**

**Fresh Mango (one, peeled and diced):** Infuse the smoothie with the exotic sweetness of mango, offering a rich source of vitamins A and C.

**Fresh Spinach Leaves (two cups):** Add a vibrant burst of green goodness with fresh spinach, providing essential nutrients like iron, folate, and antioxidants.

**Banana (one ripe):** Introduce natural sweetness and creaminess with a ripe banana, contributing potassium, vitamins, and energy.

**Greek Yoghurt (1/2 cup):** Provide a creamy texture and additional nutrients with Greek yoghurt, supplying probiotics for gut health.

**Chia Seeds (one tablespoon):** Boost the nutritional content with chia seeds, delivering omega-3 fatty acids, fibre, and a subtle crunch.

**Coconut Water (one cup):** Create a hydrating and tropical base with coconut water, offering a light and refreshing essence.

**Method of Preparation:**

To prepare the "Mango Green Revitalizer Blend," follow these simple steps:

**Prepare Ingredients:** Peel and dice fresh mango, measure spinach leaves, peel the ripe banana, and gather Greek yoghurt, chia seeds, and coconut water.

**Blending Process:** In a blender, combine the diced mango, fresh spinach leaves, ripe banana, Greek yoghurt, chia seeds, and coconut water.

**Blend Until Smooth:** Blend the ingredients until achieving a smooth and velvety consistency, ensuring the mango and spinach are fully incorporated.

**Adjust Consistency (Optional):** If a thicker or thinner consistency is required, adjust by adding more coconut water or water and blend again.

**Serve and Enjoy:** Pour the Mango Green Revitalizer Blend into glasses, perhaps over ice for an extra refreshing touch. Garnish with a mango slice or a sprinkle of chia seeds for visual appeal.

**Benefits:**

**Mango's Tropical Nutrients:** Mangoes provide a tropical burst of vitamins A and C, promoting immune health and skin vitality.

**Leafy Goodness from Spinach:** Spinach contributes iron, folate, and antioxidants, supporting overall well-being.

**Natural Sweetness and Potassium:** The ripe banana adds natural sweetness and potassium, aiding muscle function and heart health.

**Probiotics from Greek Yoghurt:** Greek yoghurt introduces probiotics, promoting a healthy gut microbiome and aiding digestion.

**Omega-3 and Fibre from Chia Seeds:** Chia seeds offer omega-3 fatty acids and fibre, supporting heart health and digestive well-being.

**Hydration with Coconut Water:** Coconut water provides a hydrating and electrolyte-rich base, contributing to overall hydration.

Indulge in the tropical allure of the "Mango Green Revitalizer Blend," a smoothie designed to transport you to a paradise of flavours and provide your body with a nourishing boost. Celebrate the fusion of mango and spinach as you embark on a journey of revitalization and well-being.

# 34

## Sunset Glow Sweet Potato Detox Fusion

Embark on a journey of vibrant nourishment with the "Sunset Glow Sweet Potato Detox Fusion,"a harmonious blend that unites the earthy sweetness of sweet potatoes, the tropical allure of mango, and the vibrant richness of beets. This smoothie is a celebration of flavours and nutrients, offering a symphony of colours and wellness benefits. Indulge in the captivating hues of the sunset as you sip on this detox fusion, where wholesome ingredients converge to create a delicious and revitalizing elixir.

**Ingredients:**

**Sweet Potatoes (one cup, cooked and peeled):** Harness the nutrient-rich goodness of sweet potatoes, providing a rich source of vitamins, minerals, and antioxidants.

**Mango (one cup, diced):** Introduce tropical sweetness with mango, adding vitamins A and C, as well as natural sugars for a delightful taste.

**Beets (one small, peeled and diced):** Enhance the smoothie's colour and nutritional profile with beets, offering antioxidants and potential benefits for heart health.

**Greek Yogurt (1/2 cup):** Provide a creamy texture and additional nutrients with Greek yoghurt, supplying probiotics for gut health.

**Chia Seeds (one tablespoon):** Boost the nutritional content with chia seeds, delivering omega-3 fatty acids, fibre, and a subtle crunch.

**Almond Milk (one cup):** Create a smooth and dairy-free base with almond milk, offering a nutty flavour and essential nutrients.

**Method of preparation:**

To prepare the "Sunset Glow Sweet Potato Detox Fusion," follow these simple steps:

**Prepare Ingredients:** Cook and peel the sweet potatoes, dice the mango, peel and dice the beets, and measure Greek yoghurt, chia seeds, and almond milk.

**Blending Process:** In a blender, combine the cooked and peeled sweet potatoes, diced mango, peeled and diced beets, Greek yoghurt, chia seeds, and almond milk.

**Blend Until Smooth:** Blend the ingredients until achieving a smooth and velvety consistency, ensuring the sweet potato and beets are fully incorporated.

**Adjust Consistency (Optional):** If a thicker or thinner consistency is desired, adjust by adding more almond milk or water and blend again.

**Serve and Enjoy:** Pour the Sunset Glow Sweet Potato Detox Fusion into glasses, perhaps over ice, for an extra refreshing touch. Garnish with a slice of mango or a sprinkle of chia seeds for visual appeal.

**Benefits:**

**Nutrient-Rich Sweet Potatoes:** Sweet potatoes provide a rich source of vitamins A and C, potassium, and dietary fibre, promoting overall health.

**Tropical Mango Goodness:** Mango contributes natural sweetness, along with vitamins A and C, supporting immune health and providing a tropical flavour.

**Beet Antioxidant Power:** Beets offer antioxidants and potential benefits for heart health, enhancing the smoothie's nutritional profile.

**Probiotics from Greek Yoghurt:** Greek yoghurt introduces probiotics, promoting a healthy gut microbiome and aiding digestion.

**Omega-3 and Fibre from Chia Seeds:** Chia seeds offer omega-3 fatty acids and fibre, supporting heart health and digestive well-being.

**Dairy-Free Nutrients:** Almond milk provides a dairy-free base with essential nutrients like vitamin E and calcium.

Immerse yourself in the captivating allure of the "Sunset Glow Sweet Potato Detox Fusion," a smoothie that not only tantalizes your taste buds but also infuses your body with the nourishing benefits of sweet potatoes, mango, and beets. Celebrate the beauty of this nutrient-packed fusion as you sip your way to a revitalized and refreshed state.

# 35

## Tropical Refresh Cleanse Blend

Embark on a revitalizing journey with the “Tropical Refresh Cleanse Blend,” a vibrant and refreshing smoothie that harmoniously combines the crisp essence of cucumber, the creamy sweetness of banana, and the tropical delight of pineapple. This enticing blend is a celebration of flavours and wellness, offering a burst of hydration and nourishment. Immerse yourself in the tropical oasis of this smoothie, where the invigorating properties of its ingredients come together to create a revitalizing elixir.

**Ingredients:**

**Cucumber (one medium, peeled and sliced):** Infuse the smoothie with crisp hydration and a mild flavour, providing a refreshing base.

**Banana (one, ripe):** Add natural sweetness and creaminess with a ripe banana, offering potassium, vitamins, and energy.

**Pineapple (ne cup, diced):** Introduce a tropical flair with diced pineapple, providing a rich source of vitamins, antioxidants, and enzymes.

**Greek Yoghurt (1/2 cup):** Provide a creamy texture and additional nutrients with Greek yoghurt, supplying probiotics for gut health.

**Chia Seeds (one tablespoon):** Boost the nutritional content with chia seeds, delivering omega-3 fatty acids, fibre, and a subtle crunch.

**Coconut Water (one cup):** Create a hydrating and tropical base with coconut water, offering electrolytes and a hint of natural sweetness.

**Method of preparation:**

To prepare the "Tropical Refresh Cleanse Blend," follow these simple steps:

**Prepare Ingredients:** Peel and slice cucumber, peel the ripe banana, dice pineapple, and measure Greek yoghurt, chia seeds, and coconut water.

**Blending Process:** In a blender, combine the sliced cucumber, peeled banana, diced pineapple, Greek yoghurt, chia seeds, and coconut water.

**Blend Until Smooth:** Blend the ingredients until achieving a smooth and velvety consistency, ensuring the cucumber and pineapple are fully incorporated.

**Adjust Consistency (Optional):** If a thicker or thinner consistency is required, adjust by adding more coconut water or water and blend again.

**Serve and Enjoy:** Pour the Tropical Refresh Cleanse Blend into glasses, perhaps over ice for an extra refreshing touch. Garnish with a pineapple slice or a sprinkle of chia seeds for visual appeal.

**Benefits:**

**Hydrating Cucumber Base:** Cucumber provides crisp hydration, contributing to overall fluid intake and promoting skin health.

**Potassium from Banana:** Banana adds natural sweetness and potassium, supporting muscle function and heart health.

**Vitamins and Enzymes in Pineapple:** Pineapple offers a rich source of vitamins, antioxidants, and enzymes, potentially aiding digestion.

**Probiotics from Greek Yogurt:** Greek yoghurt introduces probiotics, promoting a healthy gut microbiome and aiding digestion.

**Omega-3 and Fibre from Chia Seeds:** Chia seeds offer omega-3 fatty acids and fibre, supporting heart health and digestive well-being.

**Electrolytes in Coconut Water:** Coconut water provides a hydrating base with electrolytes, refreshing the body and enhancing natural hydration.

Indulge in the tropical delight of the "Tropical Refresh Cleanse Blend," a smoothie designed to invigorate your senses and infuse your body with the revitalizing benefits of cucumber, banana, and pineapple. Embrace the tropical oasis with every sip and celebrate the fusion of flavours that elevate your well-being.

# 36

## Papaya Passion Fruit Symphony Smoothie

Embark on a tantalizing journey of tropical indulgence with the "Papaya Passion Fruit Symphony Smoothie." This vibrant concoction isn't just a fusion of exotic flavours; it's a harmonious blend of nutrient-packed ingredients that transport your taste buds to a blissful paradise. Join us in unravelling the lush goodness of papaya and passion fruit, crafting a symphony of taste and well-being that will leave you refreshed and revitalized.

**Ingredients:**

**Papaya:** Brimming with vitamins, fibre, and enzymes, papaya not only tantalizes your taste buds but also supports digestion and provides a burst of tropical goodness.

**Passion Fruit:** A true tropical gem, passion fruit contributes a unique flavour profile while delivering antioxidants and immune-boosting properties.

**Greek Yoghurt:** Creamy Greek yoghurt adds a luscious texture to the smoothie while also providing probiotics for gut health and protein boost.

**Honey:** A touch of natural sweetness from honey enhances the overall taste and brings additional antioxidants and potential anti-inflammatory benefits.

**Coconut Water:** The hydrating power of coconut water not only complements the tropical theme but also replenishes electrolytes for a revitalizing experience.

**Method of preparation:**

Indulge in the preparation of the "Papaya Passion Fruit Symphony Smoothie" with these simple steps:

**Prepare Ingredients:** Peel and dice papaya, scoop out the passion fruit seeds and gather Greek yoghurt, honey, and coconut water.

**Blend to Perfection:** In a blender, blend the papaya, passion fruit seeds, Greek yoghurt, honey, and coconut water. Blend until you achieve a smooth and velvety consistency.

**Adjust Texture:** If needed, adjust the texture by adding more coconut water for a lighter feel or Greek yoghurt for a creamier texture.

**Serve Chilled:** Pour the symphony of flavours into a glass filled with ice cubes for an extra refreshing touch. Savour the tropical delight!

**Benefits:**

**Digestive Support:** Papaya's enzymes aid in digestion, while Greek yoghurt provides probiotics for a healthy gut.

**Immune Boost:** The combination of papaya and passion fruit delivers a potent dose of vitamins and antioxidants, supporting your immune system.

**Hydration and Electrolyte Replenishment:** Coconut water ensures proper hydration and replenishes electrolytes, making this smoothie perfect for a refreshing pick-me-up.

Allow the "Papaya Passion Fruit Symphony Smoothie" to transport you to a tropical oasis of well-being and flavour.

*Here's to a journey of healthful indulgence! Cheers!*

# 37

# Spirulina Sunshine Smoothie

Embark on a vibrant journey to wellness with the "Spirulina Sunshine Smoothie." This radiant elixir isn't just a burst of colour; it's a powerhouse of nutrients that brings the goodness of spirulina to your daily routine. Join us in unlocking the potential of this blue-green algae, blending it with tropical fruits to create a sunshine-infused smoothie that radiates health and vitality.

**Ingredients:**

**Spirulina Powder:** Packed with protein, vitamins, and minerals, spirulina adds a nutritional punch and vibrant colour to this smoothie.

**Pineapple:** The sweet and tangy flavour of pineapple complements the earthiness of spirulina, and contributes vitamins and digestive enzymes.

**Mango:** Rich in antioxidants and vitamins, mango adds a tropical sweetness while enhancing the smoothie's nutritional profile.

**Banana:** Creamy and naturally sweet, banana provides a smooth texture and a dose of potassium for heart health.

**Coconut Milk:** Creamy coconut milk not only enhances the tropical essence but also adds healthy fats for a satisfying and nourishing experience.

**Method of preparation:**

Craft the "Spirulina Sunshine Smoothie" with these simple steps:

**Gather Ingredients:** Peel and chop pineapple, mango, and banana. Measure the spirulina powder and coconut milk.

**Blend to Brilliance:** In a blender, combine the chopped fruits, spirulina powder, and coconut milk. Blend until you achieve a smooth and luscious consistency.

**Adjust Thickness:** If desired, adjust the thickness by adding more coconut milk for a creamier texture or ice cubes for a refreshing chill.

**Pour and Enjoy:** Pour the vibrant concoction into a glass, bask in the radiant colour, and relish the nourishing goodness of the Spirulina Sunshine Smoothie.

**Benefits:**

**Protein Boost:** Spirulina is a complete protein source, providing all essential amino acids for muscle repair and growth.

**Antioxidant Power:** Mango and pineapple contribute antioxidants, combating oxidative stress and supporting overall health.

**Nutrient-rich:** Spirulina brings a wealth of vitamins, minerals, and chlorophyll to fortify your daily nutrient intake.

**Digestive Aid:** Pineapple enzymes aid in digestion, promoting gut health and nutrient absorption.

Sip on the "Spirulina Sunshine Smoothie" and let its radiant energy uplift your senses and nourish your body.

*Here's to a sunny blend of health and delight! Cheers!*

# 38

## Dragon Fruit Dream Delight

Embark on a celestial journey of flavour and health with the "Dragon Fruit Dream Delight." This exotic smoothie is a symphony of vibrant hues and delectable taste, featuring the mystical dragon fruit as its star ingredient. Join us as we explore the enchanting world of dragon fruit, blending it with other delightful components to create a dreamy elixir that not only captivates your taste buds but also nurtures your well-being.

**Ingredients:**

**Dragon Fruit (Pitaya):** The heart of this concoction, dragon fruit, brings a burst of colour, unique texture, and an abundance of antioxidants.

**Mixed Berries:** A medley of berries, such as strawberries, blueberries, or raspberries, adds sweetness, flavour complexity, and additional antioxidants.

**Greek Yoghurt:** Creamy and rich in probiotics, Greek yoghurt provides a velvety texture while promoting gut health.

**Honey:** A touch of natural sweetness from honey complements the dragon fruit's subtle flavour, offering a delightful balance.

**Coconut Water:** Hydrating and light, coconut water enhances the tropical essence, contributing electrolytes for a refreshing experience.

**Method of preparation:**

Craft the "Dragon Fruit Dream Delight" with these simple steps:

**Prepare Dragon Fruit:** Peel and chop the dragon fruit into bite-sized cubes, appreciating its vibrant colour and texture.

**Berry Bliss:** Wash and add mixed berries to the dragon fruit, creating a delightful blend of flavours and colours.

**Yoghurt Harmony:** Spoon in Greek yoghurt for creaminess and the added benefit of gut-friendly probiotics.

**Sweet Elixir:** Drizzle honey into the mix, adjusting to your desired level of sweetness and enhancing the overall taste.

**Tropical Hydration:** Pour in coconut water, blending all ingredients until the concoction achieves a smooth and dreamy consistency.

**Pour and Revel:** Transfer the Dragon Fruit Dream Delight into a glass, marvel at its enchanting appearance, and savour the blissful journey with each sip.

**Benefits:**

**Antioxidant Magic:** Dragon fruit and mixed berries provide a powerful dose of antioxidants, combating free radicals and promoting cellular health.

**Probiotic Boost:** Greek yoghurt contributes probiotics, supports a healthy gut microbiome and aids in digestion.

**Hydration Elevation:** Coconut water not only adds a tropical twist but also hydrates, providing essential electrolytes.

Indulge in the "Dragon Fruit Dream Delight" and let its celestial flavours transport you to a realm of health and delight.

*Here's to dreaming and sipping Cheers!*

# 39

# Cranberry Coconut Cascade

Embark on a refreshing journey with the "Cranberry Coconut Cascade," a tantalizing fusion of tart cranberries and creamy coconut. This vibrant smoothie invites you to indulge in a delightful symphony of flavours while reaping the health benefits of its star ingredients. Join us as we explore the tangy allure of cranberries, harmonizing with the tropical richness of coconut, creating a cascade of taste and wellness.

**Ingredients:**

**Fresh Cranberries:** Packed with antioxidants and a tangy kick, fresh cranberries bring a burst of flavour and vibrant colour to the cascade.

**Coconut Milk:** Smooth and luscious, coconut milk adds a creamy texture, while infusing the blend with the tropical essence of coconut.

**Pineapple Chunks:** Sweet and juicy pineapple chunks contribute natural sweetness, enhancing the overall flavour profile.

**Banana:** Creamy and potassium-rich, banana provides a velvety texture and complements the tartness of cranberries.

**Greek Yoghurt:** Creamy Greek yoghurt adds a touch of richness while offering probiotics for gut health.

**Method of preparation:**

Craft the "Cranberry Coconut Cascade" with these simple steps:

**Blend Cranberries:** Start by blending fresh cranberries until they form a coarse texture, releasing their vibrant juices.

**Add Coconut Milk:** Pour in coconut milk, allowing it to intertwine with the cranberry mixture, creating a smooth and creamy base.

**Pineapple Pleasure:** Toss in pineapple chunks, introducing a tropical sweetness that harmonizes with the tart cranberries.

**Banana Bliss:** Include a ripe banana for creaminess and a subtle sweetness, rounding out the flavour profile.

**Yoghurt Embrace:** Spoon in Greek yoghurt, contributing a creamy texture and fortifying the smoothie with gut-friendly probiotics.

**Blend to Cascade:** Blend all the ingredients until the cascade achieves a harmonious consistency, ensuring a balanced blend of flavours.

**Pour and Enjoy:** Transfer the Cranberry Coconut Cascade into a glass, relishing the delightful marriage of tart cranberries and creamy coconut with each sip.

**Benefits:**

**Antioxidant-Rich:** Cranberries are known for their antioxidant properties, aiding in the neutralization of free radicals.

**Gut-Friendly Probiotics:** Greek yoghurt introduces probiotics, supporting a healthy gut microbiome and digestive system.

**Tropical Hydration:** Coconut milk and pineapple not only add tropical flair but also provide hydration and essential nutrients.

Indulge in the refreshing blend of tart and creamy with the "Cranberry Coconut Cascade."

*Cheers to a delightful cascade of taste and well-being!*

# 40

## Kiwi Kale Kreation

Embark on a vibrant and nutritious journey with the "Kiwi Kale Kreation," a green symphony that combines the invigorating flavours of kiwi with the wholesome goodness of kale. This refreshing smoothie is not only a treat for your taste buds but also a nutrient-packed elixir that celebrates the health benefits of its star ingredients. Join us as we delve into the zesty allure of kiwi harmonizing with the earthy richness of kale, creating a kreation that revitalizes and nourishes.

**Ingredients:**

**Kiwi:** Packed with vitamin C and antioxidants, kiwi adds a sweet and tangy kick, infusing the smoothie with a burst of tropical flavour.

**Kale Leaves:** Nutrient-dense and rich in vitamins, kale brings an earthy and robust essence, elevating the smoothie's health profile.

**Banana:** Creamy and potassium-rich banana contributes a velvety texture while balancing the tartness of kiwi and the earthiness of kale.

**Green Apple:** Crisp and refreshing, green apple complements the overall flavour profile, adding a touch of natural sweetness.

**Chia Seeds:** Tiny powerhouses of nutrition, chia seeds introduce omega-3 fatty acids and fibre for added texture and health benefits.

**Method of Preparation:**

Craft the "Kiwi Kale Kreation" with these simple steps:

**Peel and Dice Kiwi:** Start by peeling and dicing fresh kiwi, preparing it for the blending process.

**Kale Preparation:** Remove the stems from kale leaves and chop them into manageable pieces, ensuring even blending.

**Banana Harmony:** Peel and add a ripe banana to the mix, enhancing the smoothie's creaminess.

**Apple Inclusion:** Core and chop a green apple, incorporating its crisp sweetness into the concoction.

**Chia Seed Boost:** Sprinkle chia seeds into the blend, introducing a nutritional boost and enhancing the smoothie's texture.

**Blend to Kreation:** Blend all the ingredients until they form a harmonious kreation, ensuring a well-balanced fusion of flavours.

**Pour and Revel:** Transfer the Kiwi Kale Kreation into a glass, savouring the vibrant and revitalizing combination of kiwi and kale with each sip.

**Benefits:**

**Vitamin C Boost:** Kiwi provides a substantial dose of vitamin C, supporting immune health and skin vitality.

**Nutrient-Dense Kale:** Kale contributes essential vitamins, minerals, and antioxidants, promoting overall well-being.

**Natural Fibre:** Banana, apple, and chia seeds introduce dietary fibre, aiding digestion and supporting a healthy gut.

Experience the revitalizing blend of sweet and earthy with the "Kiwi Kale Kreation."

*Cheers to a flavourful and healthful journey!*

# 41

## Pomegranate Pistachio Power

Embark on a journey of sensory delight with the "Pomegranate Pistachio Power" smoothie, where the rich and vibrant flavours of pomegranate meet the nutty goodness of pistachios. This unique blend isn't just a treat for your taste buds; it's a powerhouse of nutrition that combines antioxidant-rich pomegranate with the protein-packed allure of pistachios. Join us in exploring the harmony of these ingredients, creating a smoothie that not only tantalizes your palate but also nourishes your body with a burst of energy.

**Ingredients:**

**Pomegranate Seeds:** Bursting with antioxidants, pomegranate seeds add a sweet and tart flavour profile, along with a vibrant burst of colour.

**Pistachios:** Nutty and protein-packed, pistachios bring a satisfying crunch and a wealth of nutrients, contributing to the smoothie's power-packed appeal.

**Greek Yoghurt:** Creamy and rich in probiotics, Greek yoghurt enhances the smoothie's texture while providing a dose of gut-friendly bacteria.

**Honey:** A natural sweetener, honey complements the tartness of pomegranate, adding a touch of sweetness to balance the flavours.

**Almond Milk:** A dairy-free alternative, almond milk lends a smooth consistency to the smoothie, ensuring a delightful and nutritious blend.

**Method of preparation:**

Preapare the "Pomegranate Pistachio Power" with these simple steps:

**Extract Pomegranate Seeds:** Begin by extracting the seeds from a fresh pomegranate and collecting them to use in the smoothie.

**Pistachio Preparation:** Shell and crush pistachios, preparing them to infuse the smoothie with their nutty essence.

**Yoghurt Harmony:** Scoop Greek yoghurt into the blend, which introduces creaminess and the benefits of probiotics.

**Sweeten with Honey:** Add a drizzle of honey to sweeten the smoothie, ensuring a well-balanced flavour profile.

**Blend to Perfection:** Blend all the ingredients until they form a smooth and velvety concoction, achieving the desired consistency.

**Pour and Enjoy:** Transfer the Pomegranate Pistachio Power into a glass, savouring the delightful combination of sweet, tart, and nutty flavours.

**Benefits:**

**Antioxidant Boost:** Pomegranate is rich in antioxidants that combat free radicals, promoting overall health and well-being.

**Protein-Packed Pistachios:** Pistachios provide a protein boost, supporting muscle health and satiety.

**Probiotic Goodness:** Greek yoghurt contributes probiotics, fostering a healthy gut microbiome.

**Natural Sweetening:** Honey adds sweetness with additional benefits like antibacterial properties and soothing qualities.

Indulge in the luscious blend of "Pomegranate Pistachio Power" for a flavourful and energizing experience.

*Cheers to a delightful and healthful journey!*

# 42

## Green Bliss Delight with Paneer

Embark on a journey of wholesome indulgence with the "Green Bliss Delight," a harmonious blend of verdant greens and the richness of paneer. This smoothie is not just a feast for the senses; it's a celebration of flavours, textures, and nourishing ingredients. Join us as we explore the fusion of nutrient-packed greens and the creamy goodness of paneer, creating a delightful concoction that promises both satisfaction and vitality.

**Ingredients:**

**Spinach:** Packed with iron and nutrients, spinach forms the vibrant green base of this blissful smoothie.

**Kale:** Known for its robust nutritional profile, kale adds depth and richness to the blend, contributing antioxidants and vitamins.

**Paneer (Cottage Cheese):** Creamy and protein-rich, paneer brings a velvety texture and satiating quality to the smoothie.

**Avocado:** Adding a dose of healthy fats, avocado contributes to the smooth and luscious consistency of the blend.

**Banana:** Offering natural sweetness and creaminess, banana enhances the overall flavour while providing energy-boosting carbohydrates.

**Almond Milk:** A dairy-free alternative, almond milk ensures a silky texture and complements the nutty undertones of paneer.

**Method of preparation:**

Craft the "Green Bliss Delight with Paneer" using these simple steps:

**Leafy Greens Harmony:** Combine spinach and kale in a blender, creating a nutrient-rich green base.

**Creamy Paneer Addition:** Introduce chunks of paneer into the blend, ensuring a velvety and satisfying texture.

**Avocado Elegance:** Add the creamy goodness of avocado to enhance the smoothie's richness.

**Banana Sweetness:** Incorporate a ripe banana for natural sweetness and a smooth consistency.

**Almond Milk Fusion:** Pour almond milk into the blender, creating a silky and well-balanced amalgamation.

**Blend to Perfection:** Blend all the ingredients until they form a smooth and luxurious concoction, achieving the desired consistency.

**Pour and Enjoy:** Transfer the Green Bliss Delight with Paneer into a glass, relishing the fusion of creamy, green goodness.

**Benefits:**

**Protein-Packed Paneer:** Paneer contributes protein, supports muscle health and provides a feeling of fullness.

**Nutrient-rich greens:** Spinach and kale offer a powerhouse of vitamins, minerals, and antioxidants for overall well-being.

**Healthy Fats from Avocado:** Avocado brings heart-healthy monounsaturated fats, supporting cardiovascular health.

**Satisfying and Energizing:** The combination of protein, healthy fats, and natural sugars from bananas provides sustained energy.

Indulge in the luxurious "Green Bliss Delight with Paneer" for a wholesome and invigorating experience.

*Cheers to a delightful and healthful journey!*

# 43

## Paneer Paradise Fusion

Embark on a culinary odyssey with the "Paneer Paradise Fusion", a symphony of flavours that merges the rich creaminess of paneer with an eclectic blend of vibrant ingredients. This fusion smoothie isn't just a delightful concoction; it's a celebration of textures, aromas, and the wholesome goodness of paneer. Join us as we explore the indulgent union of this Indian cheese with exotic fruits, creating a paradise of taste and nutrition.

**Ingredients:**

**Paneer (Cottage Cheese):** The star of this fusion, paneer brings its velvety texture and protein-packed richness.

**Mango:** Adding a tropical twist, ripe mango contributes sweetness and a luscious consistency to the blend.

**Pineapple:** Infusing a burst of citrusy sweetness, pineapple complements the creamy notes of paneer.

**Coconut Milk:** Enhancing the tropical essence, coconut milk provides a velvety texture and a hint of exotic flavour.

**Honey:** A touch of natural sweetness, honey brings its golden richness to balance the flavours.

**Mint Leaves:** Fresh mint leaves add a refreshing and aromatic element, elevating the overall experience.

**Method of Preparation:**

Prepare the "Paneer Paradise Fusion" using these simple steps:

**Paneer Perfection:** Start by blending chunks of paneer to achieve a smooth and creamy consistency.

**Tropical Symphony:** Introduce ripe mango chunks and pineapple slices into the blender, creating a tropical medley.

**Coconut Infusion:** Pour coconut milk into the blend, ensuring a velvety and luxurious texture.

**Sweet Elegance:** Add honey for a touch of natural sweetness, balancing the flavours harmoniously.

**Minty Freshness:** Toss in fresh mint leaves to infuse a refreshing and aromatic element.

**Blend to Paradise:** Blend all the ingredients until they form a smooth and paradisiacal fusion, achieving the desired consistency.

**Pour and Savour:** Transfer the Paneer Paradise Fusion into a glass, indulging in the luscious and exotic symphony.

**Benefits:**

**Protein Powerhouse:** Paneer contributes a substantial amount of protein, supports muscle health and satiety.

**Tropical Nutrients:** Mango and pineapple bring a wealth of vitamins, minerals, and antioxidants for overall well-being.

**Creamy Coconut Goodness:** Coconut milk adds healthy fats, providing a creamy texture and promoting heart health.

**Refreshing Mint:** Mint leaves offer a burst of freshness, aiding digestion and adding a delightful twist to the fusion.

Immerse yourself in the delectable "Paneer Paradise Fusion" for a taste journey that transcends culinary boundaries.

*Cheers to a fusion of flavours and a healthful indulgence!*

# 44

## Berry Paneer Burst

Embark on a journey of delightful flavour fusion with the "Berry Paneer Burst," a captivating blend that harmonizes the lusciousness of berries with the creamy richness of paneer. This smoothie isn't just a tantalizing treat for your taste buds; it's a celebration of textures, colours, and wholesome ingredients. Join us as we explore the union of vibrant berries and the velvety essence of paneer, creating a burst of exquisite flavours that promises both satisfaction and nourishment.

**Ingredients:**

**Mixed Berries (Strawberries, Blueberries, Raspberries):** Packed with antioxidants and vitamins, these berries contribute a burst of sweetness and vibrant hues.

**Paneer (Cottage Cheese):** The creamy and protein-rich paneer adds a luxurious texture, elevating the smoothie's overall richness.

**Greek Yoghurt:** Bringing a tangy twist and additional creaminess, Greek yoghurt complements the berries and paneer beautifully.

**Honey:** A touch of natural sweetness, honey enhances the flavour profile while offering its own array of health benefits.

**Almond Milk:** Ensuring a silky and dairy-free base, almond milk brings a nutty undertone that complements the paneer and berries.

**Method of preparation:**

Craft the "Berry Paneer Burst" using these simple steps:

**Berry Bliss Fusion:** Combine a generous handful of mixed berries in a blender, creating a vibrant and antioxidant-rich base.

**Creamy Paneer Addition:** Introduce chunks of paneer into the blend, ensuring a velvety and satisfying texture.

**Greek Yoghurt Harmony:** Add a dollop of Greek yoghurt to enhance the creaminess and infuse a delightful tang.

**Sweet Honey Accent:** Drizzle honey into the blend, providing a natural sweetness that elevates the overall flavour profile.

**Almond Milk Symphony:** Pour almond milk into the blender, creating a smooth and well-balanced amalgamation of flavours.

**Blend to Perfection:** Blend all the ingredients until they form a smooth and luxurious concoction, achieving the desired consistency.

**Pour and Enjoy:** Transfer the Berry Paneer Burst into a glass, relishing the burst of flavours and the creamy indulgence.

**Benefits:**

**Antioxidant Powerhouse:** Mixed berries bring a wealth of antioxidants, supporting overall health and well-being.

**Protein-Rich Paneer:** Paneer contributes protein, aiding in muscle health and providing a sense of satiety.

**Gut-Friendly Yoghurt:** Greek yoghurt introduces probiotics for gut health and support digestion.

**Natural Sweetness of Honey:** Honey adds sweetness without refined sugars, offering its own array of health benefits.

Indulge in the delectable "Berry Paneer Burst" for a delightful and healthful experience.

*Cheers to the burst of flavours and nourishment!*

# 45

## Tropical Veggie Infusion with Paneer

Embark on a tropical journey of vibrant flavours and nourishment with the "Tropical Veggie Infusion," a delightful blend enriched with the goodness of paneer. This smoothie isn't just a taste bud tantalizer; it is a symphony of tropical fruits, vegetables, and the creamy delight of paneer. Join us as we explore a fusion of tropical sensations and wholesome ingredients, creating a refreshing elixir that promises both indulgence and well-being.

**Ingredients:**

**Mango:** Transport your taste buds to the tropics with the sweet and juicy essence of mango, rich in vitamins and antioxidants.

**Pineapple:** Add a tropical zing with pineapple, providing a burst of refreshing flavour and enzymes for digestion.

**Spinach:** Infuse the smoothie with nutrient-packed spinach, offering a dose of vitamins, minerals, and antioxidants.

**Paneer (Cottage Cheese):** Elevate the creaminess and protein content with chunks of paneer, adding a satisfying element to the blend.

**Cucumber:** Introduce crispness and hydration with cucumber, contributing a refreshing balance to the tropical mix.

**Coconut Water:** Enhance the tropical experience with the natural hydration of coconut water, providing electrolytes and a subtle sweetness.

**Method of Preparation:**

Craft the "Tropical Veggie Infusion with Paneer" using these simple steps:

**Tropical Fruit Fusion:** Combine mango chunks and pineapple in a blender, creating a tropical fruit base.

**Nutrient-rich greens:** Add fresh spinach to the mix, incorporating vitamins and antioxidants into the infusion.

**Creamy Paneer Addition:** Introduce chunks of paneer into the blend, ensuring a velvety and satisfying texture.

**Cucumber Freshness:** Include cucumber slices for a crisp and hydrating element, balancing the sweetness of fruits.

**Coconut Water Bliss:** Pour coconut water into the blender, infusing the smoothie with tropical hydration.

**Blend to Perfection:** Blend all the ingredients until they form a smooth and luxurious concoction, achieving the desired consistency.

**Pour and Enjoy:** Transfer the Tropical Veggie Infusion with Paneer into a glass, savouring the tropical burst and creamy goodness.

**Benefits:**

**Protein-Packed Paneer:** Paneer contributes protein, supports muscle health and provides a feeling of fullness.

**Tropical Vitamin Boost:** Mango and pineapple offer a wealth of vitamins, particularly vitamin C, for immune support.

**Hydrating Coconut Water:** Coconut water provides natural electrolytes, enhances hydration and supports overall well-being.

**Nutrient-Rich Spinach:** Spinach contributes essential vitamins, minerals, and antioxidants, promoting overall health.

Indulge in the tropical paradise of "Tropical Veggie Infusion with Paneer" for a refreshing and nourishing experience.

*Cheers to a tropical delight and a healthful journey!*

# 46

## Spinach Mango Tango with Paneer Essence

Embark on a flavour-packed journey with the "Spinach Mango Tango," a vibrant and nutritious fusion that seamlessly blends the goodness of spinach, the tropical sweetness of mango, and the creamy essence of paneer. This delightful concoction is not just a dance of flavours; it's a celebration of health and indulgence. Join us as we explore the harmonious marriage of nutrient-rich greens, succulent mango, and the satisfying creaminess of paneer, creating a dance of taste and well-being.

**Ingredients:**

**Spinach:** A nutritional powerhouse, spinach forms a verdant base, providing vitamins, minerals, and antioxidants.

**Mango:** Bursting with tropical sweetness, mango adds a luscious and fruity dimension to the smoothie.

**Paneer (Cottage Cheese):** Infusing the blend with a creamy and protein-rich essence, paneer elevates the smoothie's texture.

**Banana:** Contributing to natural sweetness and creaminess, banana enhances the overall flavour profile.

**Greek Yoghurt:** Introducing a tangy and velvety component, Greek yoghurt complements the richness of paneer.

**Almond Milk:** Ensuring a smooth and liquid consistency, almond milk adds a nutty undertone to the infusion.

**Method of Preparation:**

Prepare the "Spinach Mango Tango with Paneer Essence" using these simple steps:

**Leafy Greens Base:** Blend fresh spinach to form a nutrient-packed green foundation for the smoothie.

**Mango Sweetness:** Add ripe mango chunks to the blender, infusing the blend with tropical succulence.

**Paneer Creaminess:** Incorporate chunks of paneer, ensuring a delightful and satisfying creaminess.

**Banana Smooth Consistency:** Include a ripe banana for natural sweetness and a velvety smooth texture.

**Yoghurt Harmony:** Introduce Greek yoghurt to bring a tangy and creamy balance to the blend.

**Almond Milk Fusion:** Pour almond milk into the blender, creating a silky and well-balanced amalgamation.

**Blend to Perfection:** Blend all the ingredients until they form a smooth and luxurious concoction, achieving the desired consistency.

**Pour and Revel:** Transfer the Spinach Mango Tango with Paneer Essence into a glass, savouring the dance of tropical and creamy flavours.

**Benefits:**

**Nutrient-rich greens:** Spinach provides an abundance of vitamins, minerals, and antioxidants for overall well-being.

**Tropical Mango Bliss:** Mango brings a dose of tropical sweetness along with vitamins and dietary fibre.

**Protein-Packed Paneer:** Paneer contributes protein, supports muscle health and satiety.

**Creamy Delight with Greek Yoghurt:** Greek yoghurt adds a velvety texture and a tangy dimension to the smoothie.

Dance to the tune of health and indulgence with the "Spinach Mango Tango with Paneer Essence."

*Cheers to a delightful and healthful journey!*

# 47

## Citrus Paneer Splash

Dive into a refreshing symphony of citrusy zest and creamy indulgence with the "Citrus Paneer Splash." This vibrant concoction unites the tangy brightness of citrus fruits with the luscious creaminess of paneer, creating a tropical splash that tantalizes your taste buds and nourishes your senses. Join us in savouring this delightful fusion of citrusy freshness and the velvety richness of paneer for a refreshing journey of flavour and well-being.

**Ingredients:**

**Oranges:** Infusing the smoothie with a burst of citrusy sweetness and immune-boosting vitamin C.

**Grapefruits:** Adding a tangy twist and additional citrusy goodness to the blend.

**Paneer (Cottage Cheese):** Paneer elevates the smoothie's texture and introduces a creamy and protein-rich essence.

**Banana:** Providing natural sweetness and contributing to the smooth and velvety consistency.

**Greek Yoghurt:** Bringing a tangy and velvety component that complements the richness of paneer.

**Honey:** Adding a touch of natural sweetness to balance the citrusy tartness.

**Ice Cubes:** Ensuring a refreshing chill to enhance the overall drinking experience.

**Method of preparation:**

Craft the "Citrus Paneer Splash" using these simple steps:

**Citrus Fusion:** Squeeze fresh orange and grapefruit juice into the blender for a vibrant citrus base.

**Paneer Creaminess:** Incorporate chunks of paneer to infuse a luxurious and creamy texture.

**Banana Sweetness:** Add a ripe banana for natural sweetness and a smooth consistency.

**Yoghurt Harmony:** Introduce Greek yoghurt to bring a tangy and creamy balance to the blend.

**Drizzle of Honey:** Include honey for a touch of sweetness that complements the citrusy tartness.

**Ice for Refreshment:** Drop in ice cubes to ensure a refreshing and chilled delight.

**Blend to Perfection:** Blend all the ingredients until they form a smooth and indulgent concoction.

**Pour and Enjoy:** Pour the Citrus Paneer Splash into a glass, and relish the harmonious dance of citrusy freshness and creamy delight.

**Benefits:**

**Citrus Vitamin Boost:** Oranges and grapefruits provide a rich source of vitamin C, supporting immune health.

**Protein-Packed Paneer:** Paneer contributes protein, fostering muscle health and satiety.

**Creamy Bliss with Greek Yoghurt:** Greek yoghurt adds a velvety texture and a tangy dimension to the smoothie.

**Natural Sweetness:** Bananas and honey offer natural sweetness without the need for added sugars.

Drench your senses in the invigorating "Citrus Paneer Splash" – a delightful fusion of citrus vibrancy and creamy indulgence.

*Cheers to a refreshing and healthful journey!*

# 48

## Kiwi Kale Joy

Embark on a journey of vibrant nourishment with the "Kiwi Kale Joy," a harmonious blend of wholesome ingredients that promises a delightful burst of flavours and nourishing goodness. This invigorating smoothie combines the unique tartness of kiwi, the robust earthiness of kale, and the creamy richness of paneer, creating a symphony of tastes that dance on your palate. Let's dive into the rejuvenating experience of the "Kiwi Kale Joy" and discover the vitality that each sip brings.

**Ingredients:**

**Kiwi:** Infusing a tangy and exotic sweetness that defines the distinct character of the smoothie.

**Kale:** Provides a nutritional powerhouse with its earthy flavour and a spectrum of vitamins and minerals.

**Paneer (Cottage Cheese):** Adds a velvety richness and protein-packed creaminess to elevate the smoothie.

**Banana:** Contributes natural sweetness and a smooth consistency to balance the flavours.

**Greek Yoghurt:** Introduces a tangy and velvety component that complements the creaminess of paneer.

**Honey:** Offers a touch of natural sweetness to enhance the overall flavour profile.

**Ice Cubes:** Ensures a refreshing chill that amplifies the enjoyment of each sip.

**Method of preparation:**

Craft the "Kiwi Kale Joy" with these simple steps:

**Kiwi Extravaganza:** Peel and chop fresh kiwi, tossing it into the blender for a burst of exotic sweetness.

**Kale Green Goodness:** Add fresh kale leaves, ensuring a nutrient-packed green boost to the smoothie.

**Paneer Elegance:** Incorporate chunks of paneer, infusing a luxurious and creamy texture to the blend.

**Banana Harmony:** Introduce a ripe banana for natural sweetness and a velvety consistency.

**Yoghurt Silhouette:** Blend in Greek yoghurt to bring a tangy and creamy balance to the concoction.

**Drizzle of Honey:** Add honey for a touch of sweetness that harmonizes with the overall flavour profile.

**Ice for Refreshment:** Drop in ice cubes to ensure a refreshing and chilled delight.

**Blend to Perfection:** Blend all the ingredients until they form a smooth and joyous symphony of flavours.

**Pour and Enjoy:** Pour the Kiwi Kale Joy into a glass, relishing the vibrant interplay of kiwi, kale, and creamy paneer.

**Benefits:**

**Vitamin C Boost:** Kiwi offers a potent dose of vitamin C, supporting immune health.

**Nutrient-rich kale:** Kale brings an abundance of vitamins, minerals, and antioxidants to the mix.

**Protein-Packed Paneer:** Paneer enriches the smoothie with protein for sustained energy and satiety.

**Creamy Harmony with Greek Yoghurt:** Greek yoghurt adds a velvety texture and a tangy dimension to the blend.

Savour the "Kiwi Kale Joy" – a captivating blend of exotic sweetness, green vitality, and creamy delight.

*Cheers to a joyous and healthful journey!*

# 49

## Pomegranate Protein Boost

Elevate your vitality with the "Pomegranate Protein Boost," a luscious blend that marries the bold flavours of pomegranate with the creamy richness of protein-packed paneer. This invigorating smoothie isn't just a tantalizing treat for your taste buds; it's a powerhouse of nutrients designed to fuel your day with energy and nourishment. Join us on a flavourful journey as we explore the vibrant synergy of pomegranate and paneer, creating a smoothie that indulges your senses while providing essential protein benefits.

**Ingredients:**

- **Pomegranate Seeds:** Packed with antioxidants, pomegranate seeds infuse the smoothie with a burst of sweet and tangy flavour.
- **Paneer (Cottage Cheese):** Silently contributes to the creaminess and protein density without stealing the spotlight.
- **Banana:** Providing natural sweetness and a smooth consistency to balance the overall flavour profile.
- **Greek Yoghurt:** Introduces a velvety texture and a tangy note that complements the richness of paneer.
- **Chia Seeds:** Adding a nutritional punch with omega-3 fatty acids, fibre, and a subtle crunch.
- **Honey:** A touch of natural sweetness to enhance the flavour harmony.

**Ice Cubes:** Ensures a refreshing chill that enhances the overall enjoyment.

**Method of preparation:**

Craft the "Pomegranate Protein Boost" with the following simple steps:

**Pomegranate Extravaganza:** Extract the vibrant seeds of fresh pomegranate, infusing the smoothie with antioxidants.

**Paneer Elegance:** Incorporate chunks of paneer for a creamy texture and a protein-packed boost.

**Banana Harmony:** Add a ripe banana for natural sweetness and a velvety consistency.

**Yoghurt Silhouette:** Blend in Greek yoghurt to bring a smooth and tangy balance to the concoction.

**Chia Seed Enrichment:** Sprinkle chia seeds for added nutritional benefits and a delightful crunch.

**Drizzle of Honey:** Introduce honey to elevate the sweetness and complement the overall flavour profile.

**Ice for Refreshment:** Drop in ice cubes to ensure a refreshing and chilled delight.

**Blend to Perfection:** Blend all the ingredients until they form a smooth and protein-rich elixir.

**Pour and Enjoy:** Pour the Pomegranate Protein Boost into a glass, relishing the harmonious fusion of pomegranate and protein-packed paneer.

**Benefits:**

**Protein Powerhouse:** Paneer silently contributes a protein boost for muscle support and sustained energy.

**Antioxidant Bliss:** Pomegranate seeds bring a burst of antioxidants to combat oxidative stress.

**Nutrient-Dense Chia Seeds:** Chia seeds enrich the smoothie with omega-3 fatty acids, fibre, and essential nutrients.

**Creamy Harmony with Greek Yoghurt:** Greek yoghurt adds a velvety texture and a tangy dimension to the blend.

Indulge in the "Pomegranate Protein Boost" – a delightful union of antioxidant-rich pomegranate and protein-packed paneer.

*Cheers to a flavourful and healthful journey!*

# 50

## Avocado Spinach Bliss

Embark on a journey of nourishment with the "Avocado Spinach Bliss," a heavenly fusion of creamy avocado, nutrient-packed spinach, and the protein-rich indulgence of paneer. This wholesome smoothie is not just a treat for your taste buds; it's a symphony of flavours and nutrients designed to uplift your senses and provide a burst of healthful benefits. Join us in savouring the delicate balance of avocado, spinach, and the subtle richness of paneer, creating a blissful smoothie that indulges your palate and fuels your well-being.

**Ingredients:**

**Avocado:** Creamy and rich, avocado brings a velvety texture and healthy monounsaturated fats to the blend.

**Spinach:** Packed with essential vitamins and minerals, spinach adds a vibrant green hue and nutrient density.

**Paneer (Cottage Cheese):** Silently enhances the smoothie's protein content and contributes a subtle creaminess.

**Banana:** Providing natural sweetness and contributing to the smooth consistency of the blend.

**Greek Yoghurt:** Adds a tangy note and a velvety texture that complements the overall flavour profile.

**Almond Milk:** Ensures a dairy-free and nutty undertone for a luscious, plant-powered experience.

**Chia Seeds:** Infuses the blend with omega-3 fatty acids, fibre, and a delightful crunch.

**Method of Preparation:**

Craft the "Avocado Spinach Bliss" with these simple steps:

**Avocado Elegance:** Scoop out the creamy goodness of ripe avocado, ensuring a luxurious texture.

**Spinach Symphony:** Add fresh spinach leaves for a nutrient-packed green boost and vibrant colour.

**Paneer Harmony:** Introduce chunks of paneer for a protein-rich, subtle creaminess without overtaking the flavours.

**Banana Sweetness:** Incorporate a ripe banana for natural sweetness and a velvety consistency.

**Yoghurt Unison:** Blend in Greek yoghurt for a tangy dimension that complements the richness of paneer.

**Almond Milk Addition:** Pour in almond milk to achieve a dairy-free and nutty undertone.

**Chia Seed Enrichment:** Sprinkle chia seeds for added nutritional benefits and a delightful crunch.

**Blend to Perfection:** Blend all the ingredients until they form a smooth, creamy, and nourishing elixir.

**Pour and Savour:** Pour the Avocado Spinach Bliss into a glass, relishing the harmonious fusion of avocado, spinach, and protein-packed paneer.

**Benefits:**

**Creamy Avocado Goodness:** Avocado contributes healthy monounsaturated fats for heart health and satiety.

**Nutrient-Rich Spinach:** Spinach adds essential vitamins and minerals for overall well-being.

**Protein-Packed Paneer:** Paneer subtly enhances the protein content and supports muscle health.

**Plant-Powered Almond Milk:** Almond milk provides a dairy-free and nutty base for a luscious plant-powered experience.

Indulge in the "Avocado Spinach Bliss" - a delightful marriage of creamy avocado, nutrient-packed spinach, and protein-rich paneer.

*Cheers to a flavourful and healthful journey!*

# 51

## Pineapple Paneer Paradise

Embark on a tropical escapade with the “Pineapple Paneer Paradise.” This delightful fusion of succulent pineapple and protein-rich paneer is more than a refreshing smoothie - it’s a journey to a blissful paradise of flavours and nourishment. Join us in savouring the essence of the tropics and the subtle richness of paneer, creating a smoothie that transports your taste buds to a sun-kissed haven.

**Ingredients:**

**Pineapple Chunks:** Infusing the smoothie with the tropical sweetness and vibrant flavour of fresh pineapple.

**Paneer (Cottage Cheese):** Adding a creamy and protein-packed element, seamlessly blending into the tropical symphony.

**Coconut Milk:** Introducing a luscious coconut milk base, enhancing the tropical essence and complementing the paneer’s richness.

**Banana:** Contributing natural sweetness and a smooth consistency to the blend.

**Greek Yoghurt:** Infusing a tangy and creamy note, elevating the overall texture and taste.

**Honey:** A touch of natural sweetness to harmonize the flavours and add a hint of decadence.

**Ice Cubes:** Provides a refreshing chill, reminiscent of an island breeze.

**Method of Preparation:**

Craft the "Pineapple Paneer Paradise" with these simple steps:

**Tropical Pineapple Bliss:** Add generous chunks of fresh pineapple for a burst of tropical sweetness.

**Paneer Elevation:** Incorporate paneer for its protein richness and subtle creaminess.

**Coconut Milk Oasis:** Pour in coconut milk, creating a luscious base that complements both pineapple and paneer.

**Banana Harmony:** Toss in a ripe banana for its natural sweetness and velvety texture.

**Yoghurt Luxury:** Introduce Greek yoghurt for a tangy and creamy dimension that enhances the overall mouthfeel.

**Drizzle of Honey:** Add honey to balance the flavours and add a touch of indulgence.

**Ice for the Island Breeze:** Drop in ice cubes for a refreshing chill, evoking the sensation of a tropical paradise.

**Blend to Paradise:** Blend all the ingredients until they form a smooth and heavenly concoction.

**Pour and Immerse:** Pour the Pineapple Paneer Paradise into a glass, immersing yourself in the tropical symphony.

**Benefits:**

**Tropical Bliss:** Pineapple brings a burst of tropical sweetness, transporting you to a sun-kissed paradise.

**Protein-Rich Paneer:** Silent yet powerful, paneer contributes protein for muscle support and sustained energy.

**Creamy Coconut Indulgence:** Coconut milk and Greek yoghurt create a creamy base, enhancing the overall richness.

**Nutrient-Packed Banana:** Adds natural sweetness and essential nutrients, complementing the tropical flavours.

Indulge in the "Pineapple Paneer Paradise" – a tropical haven where pineapple meets protein-rich paneer in a blissful smoothie.

*Cheers to a flavourful and healthful journey!*

# 52

# Ayurvedic Cleanse Elixir

Embark on a holistic journey of rejuvenation with the "Ayurvedic Cleanse Elixir." Rooted in ancient Ayurvedic wisdom, this elixir is crafted to cleanse not only the body but also the mind and spirit. Immerse yourself in a harmonious blend of Ayurvedic herbs and flavours, carefully curated to promote balance, vitality, and overall well-being. Join us in savouring the time-honoured practices of Ayurveda in a modern elixir that transcends cleansing to become a ritual of self-care.

**Ingredients:**

**Triphala Blend:** A combination of three potent Ayurvedic fruits - amla, haritaki, and bibhitaki - known for their cleansing properties and digestive support.

**Tulsi (Holy Basil):** Revered in Ayurveda for its adaptogenic and stress-relieving qualities, Tulsi brings a soothing and balancing element.

**Ginger Infusion:** Harnessing the anti-inflammatory and digestion-boosting powers of ginger, promoting a gentle detox.

**Turmeric Elixir:** Featuring the golden spice turmeric, celebrated for its anti-inflammatory and antioxidant benefits, supporting overall health.

**Aloe Vera Gel:** Adding a touch of soothing Aloe Vera for its healing properties and digestive support.

**Fennel Seeds:** Offering a mild, licorice-like flavour, fennel seeds aid digestion and provide a gentle cleansing effect.

**Warm Water:** Providing a hydrating base that complements the Ayurvedic herbs, promoting optimal absorption.

**Method of Preparation:**

Prepare the "Ayurvedic Cleanse Elixir" with these simple steps:

**Triphala Infusion:** Steep the triphala blend in warm water, allowing the fruits to release their cleansing properties.

**Tulsi Touch:** Add fresh or dried Tulsi leaves, infusing the elixir with their calming and adaptogenic qualities.

**Ginger Essence:** Incorporate freshly grated ginger, enhancing the elixir with its anti-inflammatory and digestive benefits.

**Turmeric Elevation:** Introduce a dash of turmeric, infusing the elixir with the golden spice's healing properties.

**Aloe Vera Addition:** Include a dollop of Aloe Vera gel, contributing to the elixir's soothing and digestive effects.

**Fennel Finale:** Sprinkle fennel seeds into the elixir, providing a mild, aromatic note and aiding digestion.

**Stir and Sip:** Mix the ingredients well and sip the Ayurvedic Cleanse Elixir mindfully, allowing its holistic essence to unfold.

**Benefits:**

**Gentle Detoxification:** Triphala, ginger, and turmeric work synergistically to support the body's natural detoxification processes.

**Digestive Harmony:** Fennel seeds and Aloe Vera contribute to a soothing and digestive-friendly elixir.

**Adaptogenic Support:** Tulsi brings adaptogenic qualities, helps the body adapt stress and promotes balance.

**Anti-Inflammatory Boost:** Ginger and turmeric lend their anti-inflammatory properties, supporting overall well-being.

Immerse yourself in the ancient wisdom of Ayurveda with the "Ayurvedic Cleanse Elixir" - a holistic elixir that cleanses not just the body but also the soul.

*Cheers to a flavourful and healthful journey!*

# 53

## Green Detox Goddess

Step into the realm of revitalization with the "Green Detox Goddess" – an elixir that embodies the essence of green goodness. Crafted with an array of nutrient-packed ingredients, this elixir is designed to cleanse, rejuvenate, and elevate your well-being. Immerse yourself in the vibrant hues of kale, the refreshing crispness of cucumber, and the nourishing creaminess of avocado, all harmonized in a symphony of flavours. Let this elixir be your guide to a revitalized and radiant you.

**Ingredients:**

**Kale Leaves (1 cup, stemmed):** Packed with vitamins and minerals, kale forms the green foundation for a nutrient-rich elixir.

**Cucumber (1/2 cup, peeled and sliced):** Refreshing cucumber adds hydration and a light, crisp note to the blend.

**Avocado (1/2):** Creamy and nutrient-dense, avocado contributes a velvety texture and healthy fats.

**Green Apple (1/2, cored and chopped):** Bringing a touch of sweetness, green apple complements the overall flavour profile.

**Lemon (1/2, juiced):** The citrusy brightness of lemon adds a zing, balancing the richness of other ingredients.

**Chlorella Powder (1 teaspoon):** A green superfood known for detoxifying properties, contributing to the elixir's cleansing nature.

**Spirulina Powder (1 teaspoon):** Another powerhouse of nutrients, spirulina enhances the elixir with its vibrant green hue and health benefits.

**Fresh Mint Leaves (1 tablespoon):** Mint introduces a refreshing and invigorating element, enlivening the palate.

**Honey or Agave Syrup (1 teaspoon, optional):** For those desire a hint of sweetness, honey or agave syrup adds a touch of indulgence.

**Water or Coconut Water (1 cup):** A hydrating base that ensures optimal blending and a smooth consistency.

**Ice Cubes (optional):** Perfect for those who prefer a chilled, refreshing elixir.

**Method of Preparation:**

**Prepare Ingredients:** Wash, peel, and chop the fruits and vegetables as needed.

**Blending Time:** In a blender, combine kale, cucumber, avocado, green apple, lemon juice, chlorella powder, spirulina powder, mint leaves, and sweetener if desired.

**Liquid Harmony:** Pour in water or coconut water to facilitate blending. Add ice cubes if a chilled elixir is preferred.

**Blend to Perfection:** Blend all ingredients until smooth, ensuring a harmonious fusion of flavours.

**Serve and Savour:** Pour the Green Detox Goddess into a glass, and relish the vibrant colours and rejuvenating flavours.

**Benefits:**

**Nutrient-Packed Goodness:** A plethora of vitamins, minerals, and antioxidants from kale, avocado, and green apple.

**Detoxifying Elixir:** Chlorella and spirulina contribute to the elixir's detoxifying properties, supporting overall well-being.

**Hydration Boost:** Cucumber and coconut water provide a hydrating foundation, promoting optimal hydration.

**Digestive Refresh:** Mint adds a refreshing touch while supporting digestive comfort.

**Energizing Elements:** The combination of natural sugars, healthy fats, and nutrient-dense ingredients provides an energy boost.

Indulge in the "Green Detox Goddess" – a vibrant elixir that celebrates the essence of green vitality and rejuvenation.

*Cheers to a flavourful and healthful journey!*

# 54

## Minty Citrus Revitalizer

Embark on a revitalizing journey with the "Minty Citrus Revitalizer" – an invigorating elixir that seamlessly blends the vibrant freshness of citrus with the cool essence of mint. This concoction is not just a delightful treat for your taste buds; it's a burst of rejuvenation for your senses. Let the wholesome spinach, succulent pineapple, and zesty citrus fruits dance in harmony, while mint imparts a refreshing twist. With a touch of chia seeds, ginger, and fennel, this elixir is designed to uplift and revitalize your spirit.

**Ingredients:**

**Fresh Spinach Leaves (1 cup):** A nutrient powerhouse, spinach brings vitamins and minerals to the mix.

**Pineapple Chunks (1/2 cup):** Juicy and sweet, pineapple adds a tropical touch and a dose of Vitamin C.

**Orange (1, peeled and segmented):** The citrusy goodness of orange introduces a zesty and refreshing flavour.

**Lemon (1/2, juiced):** Lemon juice adds a tangy kick, balancing the sweetness of fruits.

**Fresh Mint Leaves (1 tablespoon):** Mint contributes a cool and invigorating element, awakening the palate.

**Chia Seeds (1 teaspoon):** These tiny powerhouses bring a dose of fibre, omega-3 fatty acids, and texture.

**Grated Ginger (1 teaspoon):** Ginger adds a subtle warmth and complements the overall flavour profile.

**Fennel Seeds (1 teaspoon):** Fennel imparts a hint of licorice-like flavour, enhancing the elixir's complexity.

**Honey or Agave Syrup (1 teaspoon, optional):** For those with a sweet tooth, a touch of honey or agave syrup can be added.

**Coconut Water (1 cup):** A hydrating base that enhances the tropical essence of the elixir.

**Ice Cubes (optional):** Ideal for those who prefer a chilled and refreshing beverage.

**Method:**

**Prepare Ingredients:** Wash, peel, and chop fruits as needed.

**Blending Bliss:** In a blender, combine spinach, pineapple chunks, orange segments, lemon juice, mint leaves, chia seeds, grated ginger, fennel seeds, and sweetener if desired.

**Liquid Harmony:** Pour in coconut water to facilitate blending. Add ice cubes for a refreshing chill.

**Blend to Perfection:** Blend all ingredients until smooth, ensuring a harmonious fusion of flavours and textures.

**Serve and Savour:** Pour the Minty Citrus Revitalizer into a glass. Revel in vibrant colours and the refreshing burst of flavours.

**Benefits:**

**Nutrient-Rich Elixir:** A blend of fruits and greens provides essential vitamins, minerals, and antioxidants.

**Hydration Boost:** Coconut water serves as a hydrating base, replenishing electrolytes and promoting hydration.

**Digestive Support:** Ginger and fennel seeds may aid in digestion, providing a soothing touch.

**Omega-3 Goodness:** Chia seeds bring omega-3 fatty acids, contributing to heart health and overall well-being.

Indulge in the “Minty Citrus Revitalizer” – a rejuvenating elixir that harmonizes freshness, flavour, and vitality.

*Cheers to a flavourful and healthful journey!*

# 55

## Turmeric Tonic Twist

Embark on a journey of wellness with the "Turmeric Tonic Twist," a tantalizing blend that marries the golden hues of turmeric with the tropical sweetness of pineapple and the creaminess of coconut milk. This nourishing elixir is not just a feast for your taste buds but a holistic tonic enriched with the anti-inflammatory prowess of turmeric and the goodness of wholesome ingredients. Let the vibrant banana, the exotic pineapple, and the warm spices dance together in a concoction designed to rejuvenate and delight.

**Ingredients:**

**Coconut Milk (1 cup):** A luscious and creamy base that complements the tropical flavours.

**Banana (1, peeled):** Adds natural sweetness, creaminess, and a boost of potassium.

**Pineapple Chunks (1/2 cup):** Brings a burst of tropical sweetness and Vitamin C.

**Turmeric Powder (1 teaspoon):** The star ingredient is known for its anti-inflammatory properties.

**Cinnamon (1/2 teaspoon):** A warm and aromatic spice that enhances the overall flavour profile.

**Chia Seeds (1 tablespoon):** Tiny powerhouses that add texture and contribute to the nutrient content.

**Honey or Maple Syrup (one teaspoon, optional):** For those who prefer a touch of sweetness.

**Black Pepper (A pinch):** Enhances the absorption of turmeric, amplifying its benefits.

**Ice Cubes (optional):** Ideal for those who enjoy a refreshingly chilled beverage.

**Method of Preparation:**

**Prepare Ingredients:** Gather, peel, and chop fruits as needed.

**Blending Brilliance:** In a blender, combine coconut milk, peeled banana, pineapple chunks, turmeric powder, cinnamon, chia seeds, sweetener if desired, and a pinch of black pepper.

**Blend to Perfection:** Blend all the ingredients until you achieve a smooth and velvety consistency.

**Sweeten to Taste:** Adjust sweetness with honey or maple syrup if desired. Blend briefly.

**Chill and Serve:** If you desire, add ice cubes and blend briefly for a refreshing chill. Pour into a glass and savour the vibrant hues.

**Benefits:**

**Anti-Inflammatory Elixir:** Turmeric is renowned for its anti-inflammatory properties, promoting overall well-being.

**Nutrient-Rich Goodness:** A medley of fruits and chia seeds provides essential vitamins, minerals, and fibre.

**Digestive Support:** Chia seeds contribute to digestive health, offering a delightful crunch.

Sip on the "Turmeric Tonic Twist" - a vibrant elixir that fuses the goodness of turmeric, tropical flavours, and wholesome ingredients.

*Here's to a flavourful and healthful journey!*

# 56

## Cleansing Herb Fusion

Embark on a revitalizing journey with the "Cleansing Herb Fusion," a green elixir crafted to cleanse and invigorate your body. This fusion of kale, cucumber, parsley, and other cleansing herbs is not just a delightful beverage; it's a nutrient-packed powerhouse designed to support detoxification and boost overall well-being. Let the earthy kale, crisp cucumber, and zesty lemon harmonize with the herbaceous notes of cilantro and dandelion, creating a fusion that refreshes from within.

**Ingredients:**

**Kale Leaves (one cup, stemmed):** Packed with vitamins and minerals, kale forms the nutrient-rich base of this cleansing elixir.

**Cucumber (1, peeled and sliced):** Known for its hydrating properties, cucumber adds a refreshing and crisp element.

**Parsley Leaves (1/2 cup):** A vibrant herb that contributes to the detoxifying nature of the fusion.

**Lemon (1/2, juiced):** Infuses a zesty and citrusy kick, promoting digestion and adding a burst of Vitamin C.

**Cilantro Leaves (one tablespoon):** Herbaceous cilantro not only enhances the flavour but also offers its own detoxifying benefits.

**Dandelion Root Powder (one teaspoon):** Known for its potential to support liver health and detoxification.

**Spirulina Powder (one teaspoon):** A nutrient-rich algae that adds a vibrant green colour and boosts nutritional content.

**Chia Seeds (one teaspoon):** Tiny powerhouses providing omega-3 fatty acids and fibre for a satisfying texture.

**Honey or Agave Syrup (one teaspoon, optional):** For those who prefer a touch of sweetness.

**Water or Coconut Water (one cup):** The hydrating base that blends all the ingredients into a harmonious fusion.

**Ice Cubes (optional):** Perfect for those who relish a refreshing chill.

**Method of Preparation:**

**Prepare Ingredients:** Make sure kale is stemmed, cucumber is peeled and sliced, and all herbs are washed.

**Blending Brilliance:** In a blender, combine kale leaves, cucumber slices, parsley leaves, lemon juice, cilantro leaves, dandelion root powder, spirulina powder, chia seeds, sweetener if desired, and water or coconut water.

**Blend to Perfection:** Blend until all the ingredients are well incorporated, resulting in a vibrant green fusion.

**Sweeten to Taste:** Adjust sweetness with honey or agave syrup if desired. Blend briefly.

**Chill and Serve:** If desired, add ice cubes and blend briefly for a refreshing chill. Pour into a glass and relish the cleansing herb fusion.

**Benefits:**

**Detoxifying Power:** Dandelion root powder and cleansing herbs contribute to the body's natural detoxification processes.

**Nutrient-Rich Refreshment:** A blend of kale, cucumber, and spirulina provides a wealth of vitamins, minerals, and antioxidants.

**Hydration Support:** Cucumber and coconut water contribute to hydration, essential for overall well-being.

Savour the "Cleansing Herb Fusion" – a green elixir that merges the goodness of cleansing herbs into a refreshing and healthful experience.

*Here's to a flavourful and rejuvenating journey!*

# 57

## Basil Berry Herb Delight

Indulge in the symphony of flavours with the "Basil Berry Herb Delight," a vibrant concoction that combines the sweetness of mixed berries with the aromatic essence of fresh basil and the subtle earthiness of cucumber. Enriched with the goodness of Ayurvedic Triphala powder, this delightful fusion goes beyond taste, offering a plethora of health benefits. Let the tangy lemon, invigorating ginger, and optional honey or agave syrup enhance your journey to well-being.

**Ingredients:**

**Mixed Berries (strawberries, blueberries, raspberries 1 cup):** A medley of antioxidants, vitamins, and natural sweetness.

**Fresh Basil Leaves (1/2 cup):** Infuses a delightful aroma and contributes to the drink's refreshing nature.

**Cucumber (1/2, peeled and sliced):** Adds a crisp and hydrating element to the blend.

**Chia Seeds (1 tablespoon):** Tiny powerhouses of omega-3 fatty acids and fibre for added texture.

**Lemon (1/2, juiced):** Provides a zesty kick and contributes to the detoxifying nature of the elixir.

**Grated Ginger (1 teaspoon):** Adds a hint of spice and aids in digestion.

**Triphala Powder (1 teaspoon):** An Ayurvedic blend known for its holistic health benefits.

**Honey or Agave Syrup (one teaspoon, optional):** For those who prefer a touch of sweetness.

**Coconut Water or Water (1 cup):** The hydrating base that melds all the ingredients into a delightful fusion.

**Ice Cubes (optional):** Perfect for those who relish a refreshing chill.

**Method of preparation:**

**Prepare Ingredients:** Wash berries, basil leaves, and cucumber. Peel and slice the cucumber.

**Blending Brilliance:** In a blender, combine mixed berries, fresh basil leaves, cucumber slices, chia seeds, lemon juice, grated ginger, Triphala powder, sweetener (if desired), and coconut water or water.

**Blend to Perfection:** Blend until the mixture achieves a smooth and vibrant consistency.

**Sweeten to Taste:** Adjust sweetness with honey or agave syrup if desired. Blend briefly.

**Chill and Serve:** If desired, add ice cubes and blend briefly for a refreshing chill. Pour into a glass and savour the Basil Berry Herb Delight.

**Benefits:**

**Antioxidant Boost:** Mixed berries and basil contribute to the drink's antioxidant content, supporting overall health.

**Digestive Support:** Ginger aids digestion and enhances the elixir's digestive benefits.

**Ayurvedic Wellness:** Triphala powder, an Ayurvedic blend, offers holistic health benefits.

**Hydration Elevation:** Cucumber and coconut water contribute to hydration, essential for our well-being.

Delight in the "Basil Berry Herb Delight" – a flavourful infusion of nature's goodness that transcends taste, providing a holistic experience for your well-being.

*Cheers to a refreshing and healthful journey!*

# 58

# Coriander Cucumber Refresher

Embark on a journey of rejuvenation with the "Coriander Cucumber Refresher," a delightful fusion that combines the crispness of cucumber, the freshness of coriander leaves, and the sweetness of green apples. Enhanced with the zing of lemon, invigorating ginger, and the Ayurvedic goodness of Triphala powder, this refreshing elixir goes beyond quenching your thirst. Unwind and experience the hydrating and health-boosting benefits of this vibrant concoction.

**Ingredients:**

**Cucumber (one, peeled and sliced):** A hydrating base that brings a refreshing crunch.

**Fresh Coriander Leaves (one cup):** Infuses a burst of freshness and a hint of citrusy aroma.

**Green Apple (one, cored and chopped):** Adds natural sweetness and essential nutrients.

**Lemon (1/2, juiced):** Provides a citrusy kick, enhancing the drink's refreshing nature.

**Grated Ginger (one teaspoon):** Adds a subtle spiciness and aids in digestion.

**Chia Seeds (one tablespoon):** Tiny powerhouses of omega-3 fatty acids and fibre for added texture.

**Triphala Powder (one teaspoon):** An Ayurvedic blend known for holistic health benefits.

**Honey or Agave Syrup (one teaspoon, optional):** For those who prefer a touch of sweetness.

**Coconut Water or Water (one cup):** The hydrating base that melds all the ingredients into a refreshing blend.

**Ice Cubes (optional):** Perfect for those who enjoy a chilled experience.

**Method of preparation:**

**Prepare Ingredients:** Wash and peel cucumber, core and chop green apple, and gather fresh coriander leaves.

**Blending Brilliance:** In a blender, combine cucumber slices, fresh coriander leaves, green apple chunks, lemon juice, grated ginger, chia seeds, Triphala powder, sweetener if desired, and coconut water or water.

**Blend to Perfection:** Blend until the mixture achieves a smooth and invigorating consistency.

**Sweeten to Taste:** Adjust sweetness with honey or agave syrup if desired. Blend briefly.

**Chill and Serve:** If desired, add ice cubes and blend briefly for a refreshing chill. Pour into a glass and savour the Coriander Cucumber Refresher.

**Benefits:**

**Hydration Elevation:** Cucumber, coconut water, and green apple contribute to the drink's hydrating properties.

**Digestive Support:** Ginger aids digestion, enhancing the elixir's digestive benefits.

**Nutrient-Rich Refreshment:** Coriander, green apple, and lemon add essential vitamins and antioxidants.

**Ayurvedic Wellness:** Triphala powder, an Ayurvedic blend, offers holistic health benefits.

Delight in the "Coriander Cucumber Refresher" – a revitalizing blend that not only quenches your thirst but also nourishes your well-being.

*Cheers to a refreshing and healthful journey!*

# 59

# Ayurvedic Antioxidant Infusion

Embark on a journey of Ayurvedic wellness with the "Ayurvedic Antioxidant Infusion," a vibrant blend that merges the antioxidant prowess of mixed berries, the juicy burst of pomegranate seeds, and the Ayurvedic potency of amla powder. Enriched with the refreshing essence of mint, fennel seeds, and a hint of lemon, this infusion isn't just a beverage; it's a holistic experience. Immerse yourself in the harmonious balance of flavours and the revitalizing benefits of this Ayurvedic elixir.

**Ingredients:**

**Mixed Berries (one cup-blueberries, raspberries, blackberries):** A medley of antioxidants for vibrant well-being.

**Pomegranate Seeds (1/2 cup):** Juicy bursts of flavour and additional antioxidants.

**Amla Powder (one teaspoon):** Indian gooseberry, an Ayurvedic powerhouse of antioxidants.

**Fresh Mint Leaves (one tablespoon):** Adds a refreshing and aromatic touch.

**Fennel Seeds (one teaspoon):** Infuses a subtle hint of licorice flavour.

**Lemon (1/2, juiced):** Introduces a citrusy zing, enhancing the overall taste.

**Honey or Agave Syrup (one teaspoon, optional):** For those who prefer a touch of sweetness.

**Coconut Water or Water (one cup):** The hydrating base that ties all the flavours together.

**Ice Cubes (optional):** Perfect for those who enjoy a chilled experience.

**Method of Preparation:**

**Prepare Ingredients:** Wash the mixed berries thoroughly, extract pomegranate seeds and gather fresh mint leaves.

**Blending Brilliance:** In a blender, combine mixed berries, pomegranate seeds, amla powder, fresh mint leaves, fennel seeds, lemon juice, sweetener (if desired), and coconut water or water.

**Blend to Perfection:** Blend until the mixture achieves a smooth and invigorating consistency.

**Sweeten to Taste:** Adjust sweetness with honey or agave syrup if desired and blend briefly.

**Chill and Serve:** If desired, add ice cubes and blend briefly for a refreshing chill. Pour into a glass and savour the Ayurvedic Antioxidant Infusion.

**Benefits:**

**Antioxidant Boost:** Mixed berries, pomegranate, and amla powder provide a potent dose of antioxidants.

**Digestive Delight:** Fennel seeds contribute to digestive wellness.

**Refreshing Hydration:** Coconut water hydrates while adding a touch of tropical freshness.

**Ayurvedic Wellness:** Amla powder brings Ayurvedic goodness, promoting overall well-being.

Experience the holistic rejuvenation of the "Ayurvedic Antioxidant Infusion." Delight in the fusion of flavours and embrace the wellness it brings.

*Cheers to a vibrant and healthful journey!*

# 60

## Ginger Lemon Cleaning Splash

Revitalize your senses with the invigorating "Ginger Lemon Cleaning Splash." This cleansing elixir combines the zesty kick of lemon, the warmth of grated ginger, and the crispness of green apple and cucumber. Infused with the Ayurvedic potency of Triphala powder and the soothing touch of mint, this splash isn't just a drink; it's a refreshing journey towards wellness. Immerse yourself in the cleansing embrace of natural flavours and healthful benefits.

**Ingredients:**

**Grated Ginger (one tablespoon):** Infuses warmth and anti-inflammatory properties.

**Lemon (1/2, peeled and segmented):** Adds a citrusy burst and detoxifying properties.

**Green Apple (one, cored and chopped):** Offers a crisp sweetness and additional nutrients.

**Cucumber (1one, peeled and sliced):** Adds a refreshing element and hydrating properties.

**Triphala Powder (one teaspoon):** An Ayurvedic blend for digestive support and overall wellness.

**Honey or Agave Syrup (one teaspoon, optional):** Provides sweetness if desired.

**Fresh Mint Leaves (one tablespoon):** Imparts a soothing and aromatic touch.

**Water or Coconut Water (one cup):** The hydrating base that melds all the flavours.

**Ice Cubes (optional):** Enhances the refreshing experience.

**Method of Preparation:**

**Prepare Ingredients:** Peel and segment half a lemon, core and chop green apple, peel and slice cucumber and gather grated ginger, Triphala powder, honey or agave syrup, fresh mint leaves, and normal water or coconut water.

**Blending Brilliance:** In a blender, mix grated ginger, peeled and segmented lemon, chopped green apple, sliced cucumber, Triphala powder, honey or agave syrup if desired, fresh mint leaves, and normal water or coconut water.

**Blend to Perfection:** Blend until the mixture reaches a smooth and refreshing consistency.

**Sweeten to Taste:** Adjust sweetness with honey or agave syrup if desired and blend briefly.

**Chill and Serve:** If desired, add ice cubes and blend briefly for an extra refreshing splash. Pour into a glass and savour the Ginger Lemon Cleaning Splash.

**Benefits:**

**Digestive Support:** Triphala powder contributes to digestive wellness.

**Detoxification:** Lemon and ginger aid in detoxifying the body.

**Hydration and Refreshment:** Cucumber and coconut water provide hydration, while mint adds a refreshing touch.

**Antioxidant Boost:** Green apple brings additional antioxidants to the mix.

Embrace the cleansing power of the "Ginger Lemon Cleaning Splash." Let its natural flavours and healthful benefits cleanse and rejuvenate your body.

*Here's to a revitalizing and healthful journey!*

# 61

## Ayurvedic Green Radiance

Embark on a journey to radiant well-being with the "Ayurvedic Green Radiance" - a revitalizing elixir crafted with the wisdom of Ayurveda. This vibrant potion brings together the verdant goodness of spinach, the crispness of cucumber and green apple, and the herbal touch of coriander. Infused with Ayurvedic treasures like ashwagandha and spirulina, this drink isn't just a sip; it's a celebration of holistic wellness. Immerse yourself in the lush green radiance and experience the nourishment that nature has to offer.

**Ingredients:**

**Spinach Leaves (one cup):** A nutrient-dense green that contributes to overall health.

**Cucumber (1/2, peeled and sliced):** Adds a refreshing element and hydration.

**Green Apple (1/2, cored and chopped):** Brings a crisp sweetness and additional nutrients.

**Fresh Coriander Leaves (1 tablespoon):** Imparts a herbal touch and fresh flavour.

**Ashwagandha Powder (one teaspoon):** An Ayurvedic adaptogen for stress support and vitality.

**Spirulina Powder (one teaspoon):** A nutrient powerhouse rich in antioxidants and protein.

**Lemon (1/2, juiced):** Adds a zesty kick and enhances detoxification.

**Honey or Agave Syrup (one teaspoon, optional):** Provides sweetness if desired.

**Coconut Water or Water (one cup):** The hydrating base that complements the ingredients.

**Ice Cubes (optional):** Enhances the refreshing experience.

**Method of preparation:**

**Prepare Ingredients:** Peel and slice half a cucumber, core and chop half a green apple, gather spinach leaves, fresh coriander leaves, ashwagandha powder, spirulina powder, lemon for juicing, honey or agave syrup, coconut water or water, and ice cubes (if desired).

**Blending Brilliance:** In a blender, combine spinach leaves, peeled and sliced cucumber, cored and chopped green apple, fresh coriander leaves, ashwagandha powder, spirulina powder, and the juice of half a lemon.

**Liquid Harmony:** Pour in coconut water or normal water to facilitate blending. Blend until the mixture achieves a harmonious and lush green consistency.

**Sweeten to Taste:** If desired, add honey or agave syrup to sweeten the elixir. Blend briefly to incorporate.

**Chill and Serve:** Add ice cubes if you crave extra refreshment. Pour the Ayurvedic Green Radiance into a glass and relish the nourishing symphony of flavours.

**Benefits:**

**Adaptogenic Support:** Ashwagandha acts as an adaptogen and supports the body's stress response.

**Nutrient Density:** Spinach and spirulina provide a wealth of essential nutrients, promoting overall health.

**Hydration and Detoxification:** Cucumber, green apple, and lemon contribute to hydration and detoxification.

**Antioxidant Power:** Coriander and spirulina bring antioxidant benefits to the elixir.

Indulge in the Ayurvedic Green Radiance – a fusion of flavours and well-being that invites you to bask in the lush radiance of nature's gifts.

*Here's to a journey of holistic vitality and radiant health!*

# 62

## Floral Bloom Bliss Smoothie

Embark on a sensory journey with the "Floral Bloom Bliss Smoothie" - a delightful concoction inspired by the beauty and essence of flowers. This exquisite blend captures the aromatic notes and vibrant hues of floral treasures, creating a symphony of flavours that not only pleases the palate but also invigorates your senses. Immerse yourself in the gentle bloom of floral bliss, where every sip is a fragrant celebration of nature's botanical wonders.

**Ingredients:**

**Hibiscus Petals (1/4 cup):** Infuse a tart and floral note, rich in antioxidants.

**Rose Petals (1/4 cup):** Add a subtly sweet and aromatic essence to the smoothie.

**Lavender Blossoms (one tablespoon):** Imparts a soothing and fragrant undertone.

**Chamomile Flowers (one tablespoon):** Brings a mild, apple-like flavour with calming properties.

**Edible Violet Petals (one tablespoon):** Introduces a touch of vibrant colour and delicate taste.

**Mixed Berry Medley (one cup):** A blend of strawberries, blueberries, and raspberries for sweetness and antioxidants.

**Coconut Milk or Almond Milk (one cup):** Provides a creamy base for the floral infusion.

**Honey or Agave Syrup (1-2 teaspoons, optional):** Offers a hint of sweetness to balance the floral notes.

**Ice Cubes (optional):** Enhances the refreshing quality of the smoothie.

**Method of Preparation:**

**Blooming Preparation:** Gather hibiscus petals, rose petals, lavender blossoms, chamomile flowers, edible violet petals, and the mixed berry medley.

**Infusion Creation:** In a blender, combine the floral ingredients with the mixed berry medley.

**Creamy Elegance:** Pour in coconut milk or almond milk for a luscious and creamy texture.

**Optional Sweetening:** If desired, add honey or agave syrup for a touch of sweetness. Blend until the mixture achieves a harmonious consistency.

**Chill and Enjoy:** For an extra refreshing experience, add ice cubes before blending. Pour the Floral Bloom Bliss Smoothie into a glass and savour the fragrant symphony.

**Benefits:**

**Antioxidant Boost:** Hibiscus, rose, and berries contribute to the smoothie's antioxidant properties.

**Relaxing Essence:** Lavender and chamomile bring calming and soothing qualities to the blend.

**Vitamin Rich:** The mixed berry medley provides a dose of vitamins and minerals.

**Hydration and Creaminess:** Coconut milk or almond milk adds hydration and a creamy texture to the smoothie.

Indulge in the Floral Bloom Bliss Smoothie – a sensory escape into the world of blooming petals and botanical wonders.

*May each sip be a fragrant journey of floral delight!*

# 63

## Sunny Marigold Delight  Smoothie

Illuminate your senses with the "Sunny Marigold Delight Smoothie," a radiant blend inspired by the golden petals of marigold flowers. This vibrant concoction captures the essence of a sunlit garden, combining the citrusy zest of marigolds with the sweetness of tropical fruits. Let every sip transports you to a blissful realm where the warmth of the sun meets the cheerful bloom of marigolds.

**Ingredients:**

**Marigold Petals (1/4 cup):** Infuses a citrusy and slightly tangy note reminiscent of sunshine.

**Mango Chunks (one cup):** Adds a tropical sweetness and velvety texture.

**Pineapple Chunks (1/2 cup):** Enhances the fruity flavour with a tangy twist.

**Orange Juice (1/2 cup):** Introduces a burst of citrusy freshness.

**Banana (one peeled):** Provides creaminess and a subtle sweetness.

**Coconut Water (one cup):** Adds hydration and a light, refreshing base.

**Greek Yogurt (Two tablespoons, optional):** Offers a creamy texture and a touch of tanginess.

**Honey or Agave Syrup (1-2 teaspoons, optional):** Balances sweetness and enhances the overall flavour.

**Method of Preparation:**

**Marigold Infusion:** Gather marigold petals, mango chunks, pineapple chunks, and banana.

**Blending Radiance:** In a blender, combine the marigold petals, mango, pineapple, banana, and pour in the orange juice.

**Creamy Elevation:** Add coconut water and Greek yogurt if desired and blend until achieving a smooth and velvety consistency.

**Sweetening To2dxdxuch:** If more sweetness is desired, incorporate honey or agave syrup and blend briefly.

**Chill and Serve:** For a refreshing experience, refrigerate or add ice cubes before blending. Pour the Sunny Marigold Delight Smoothie into a glass and bask in the radiance.

**Benefits:**

**Citrusy Zest:** Marigold petals bring a unique citrusy flavour, uplifting the taste profile.

**Tropical Vibes:** Mango, pineapple, and banana create a tropical paradise in each sip.

**Hydration and Creaminess:** Coconut water and Greek yoghurt (optional) contribute to a light and creamy texture.

**Vitamin Boost:** The combination of fruits and marigold petals provides a boost of vitamins and antioxidants.

Embrace the golden hues and radiant flavours of the Sunny Marigold Delight Smoothie – a sunshine-filled sip that enlivens your senses with every drop!

# 64

## Hibiscus Citrus Grove Smoothie

Embark on a citrusy journey with the "Hibiscus Citrus Grove Smoothie," a refreshing blend inspired by the lively essence of a sun-kissed citrus orchard. This invigorating concoction pairs the floral notes of hibiscus with the zesty allure of citrus fruits, creating a vibrant symphony of flavours. Immerse yourself in the bright and tangy embrace of this citrus-infused delight.

**Ingredients:**

**Hibiscus Petals (1/4 cup):** Infuse a floral and slightly tart undertone.

**Citrus Trio (one orange, one grapefruit, one lemon - peeled and segmented):** Provides a zesty and refreshing citrus burst.

**Pineapple Chunks (1/2 cup):** Add tropical sweetness and a hint of acidity.

**Banana (one, peeled):** Enhances creaminess and imparts natural sweetness.

**Coconut Water (one cup):** Introduces a light and hydrating base.

**Method of Preparation:**

**Hibiscus Fusion:** Combine hibiscus petals with the citrus trio, pineapple chunks, banana, and coconut water.

**Citrus Symphony:** In a blender, blend the hibiscus-citrus mixture until it forms a vibrant and aromatic elixir.

**Creamy Texture:** Add banana for creaminess, blend until getting a smooth and delightful consistency.

**Hydration Boost:** Incorporate coconut water to enhance the overall hydration and tropical essence.

**Chill and Enjoy:** For a cool and refreshing experience, refrigerate or add ice cubes before blending. Pour the Hibiscus Citrus Grove Smoothie into a glass and relish the lively burst of citrus flavours.

**Benefits:**

**Hydration Infusion:** Coconut water and citrus fruits contribute to overall hydration, perfect for a revitalizing sip.

**Vitamin C Kick:** Citrus fruits are a powerhouse of vitamin C, boosting immune health.

**Tropical Escape:** Pineapple brings a touch of the tropics, enhancing the overall fruity profile.

Immerse yourself in the Hibiscus Citrus Grove Smoothie – a burst of citrusy bliss that transports you to a sunlit grove filled with the essence of vibrant fruits.

# 65

## Cherry Blossom Zen Elixir

Embark on a journey of tranquillity with the "Cherry Blossom Zen Elixir," a delicately crafted smoothie inspired by the serene beauty of cherry blossoms. This enchanting blend combines the sweet and slightly tart notes of cherries with a touch of floral elegance, creating a sip-worthy elixir that soothes the senses. Allow the essence of cherry blossoms to transport you to a state of blissful calmness with each delightful sip.

**Ingredients:**

**Cherries (one cup, pitted):** Infuse a natural sweetness and a hint of tartness.

**Honey (one tablespoon):** Adds a gentle sweetness that complements the cherries.

**Jasmine Green Tea (1/2 cup, chilled):** Introduces a subtle floral undertone and antioxidants.

**Almond Milk (1/2 cup):** Provides a creamy and nutty base.

**Banana (one, peeled):** Enhances creaminess and adds natural sweetness.

**Method of Preparation:**

**Cherry Blossom Infusion:** Blend pitted cherries with honey to create a luscious cherry base.

**Jasmine Harmony:** Brew jasmine green tea and let it cool before adding it to the cherry mixture.

**Creamy Silkiness:** Incorporate almond milk for a smooth and velvety texture.

**Banana Bliss:** Add a peeled banana, blend until the mixture achieves a delightful creaminess.

**Zenful Elixir:** Blend all the ingredients until you achieve a harmonious blend reminiscent of a cherry blossom garden.

**Benefits:**

**Antioxidant Boost:** Jasmine green tea contributes antioxidants and promotes overall well-being.

**Soothing Sensation:** The floral notes from jasmine tea and the sweetness of cherries create a calming elixir.

**Creamy Indulgence:** Almond milk and banana add a creamy texture, making each sip a luxurious experience.

Sip and savour the Cherry Blossom Zen Elixir, a sublime concoction that invites you to unwind and experience the serene beauty encapsulated in every drop.

# 66

## Sunflower Serenity Smoothie

Indulge in the radiance of nature with the "Sunflower Serenity Smoothie," a vibrant concoction inspired by the golden glow of sunflowers. This refreshing blend captures the essence of sunshine, combining invigorating citrus notes with the wholesome goodness of sunflower seeds. Immerse yourself in a sip that brings the warmth and positivity of a sun-kissed day.

**Ingredients:**

**Oranges (two, peeled and segmented):** Infuse a burst of citrusy freshness.

**Banana (one, peeled):** Adds creaminess and natural sweetness.

**Sunflower Seeds (two tablespoons, hulled):** Bring a nutty richness and a touch of sunshine.

**Greek Yogurt (1/2 cup):** Introduces a creamy texture and a hint of tanginess.

**Honey (one tablespoon):** Enhances sweetness and complements the overall flavour.

**Method of Preparation:**

**Citrus Radiance:** Blend peeled and segmented oranges to create a zesty citrus base.

**Banana Harmony:** Add a peeled banana, blend until a smooth consistency is achieved.

**Sunflower Embrace:** Incorporate hulled sunflower seeds, blend to infuse their nutty goodness.

**Creamy Elevation:** Introduce Greek yoghurt for a luscious and creamy texture.

**Sweet Sunshine:** Drizzle honey into the mix, blending until all components meld into a sun-kissed symphony.

**Benefits:**

**Vitamin C Boost:** Oranges contribute a generous dose of vitamin C, supporting immune health.

**Nutrient-Rich Goodness:** Sunflower seeds bring essential nutrients, including healthy fats and protein.

**Creamy Delight:** Greek yoghurt adds probiotics and a velvety smoothness to the smoothie.

Embrace the sunshine in a glass with the Sunflower Serenity Smoothie, a delightful blend that elevates your spirits and nourishes your body with each sip.

# 67

## Cherry Blossom Bliss Smoothie

Embark on a journey through the enchanting beauty of spring with the "Cherry Blossom Bliss Smoothie." This delightful concoction captures the essence of cherry blossoms in a glass, blending the sweet and floral notes of cherries with a hint of vanilla. Indulge in the delicate and uplifting flavours that blossom with each sip.

**Ingredients:**

**Cherries (one cup, pitted):** Infuse the smoothie with the sweet and vibrant essence of cherry blossoms.

**Vanilla Almond Milk (one cup):** Add a creamy texture and a touch of vanilla sweetness.

**Banana (one peeled):** Provides natural sweetness and a velvet consistency.

**Almond Butter (one tablespoon):** Introduces a nutty richness and enhances the overall flavour.

**Chia Seeds (one tablespoon):** Add a nutritional boost and a subtle crunch.

**Method of Preparation:**

**Cherry Elegance:** Blend pitted cherries to create a luscious cherry base.

**Creamy Harmony:** Pour in vanilla almond milk, blending until a creamy consistency is achieved.

**Banana Fusion:** Add a peeled banana, blend to incorporate its natural sweetness.

**Nutty Infusion:** Introduce almond butter for a delightful nutty undertone.

**Chia Elevation:** Sprinkle chia seeds into the mix, blend briefly for a nutritional boost.

**Benefits:**

**Antioxidant Rich:** Cherries bring antioxidants that promote overall health and well-being.

**Creamy Indulgence:** Vanilla almond milk and almond butter contribute to a luxurious and satisfying texture.

**Nutrient-Packed:** Chia seeds add omega-3 fatty acids, fibre, and essential nutrients.

Savour the fleeting beauty of cherry blossoms with every sip of the Cherry Blossom Bliss Smoothie – a delightful blend that transports you to a springtime haven.

# 68

## Blooming Hibiscus Bliss Smoothie

Indulge in the vibrant allure of nature with the "Blooming Hibiscus Bliss Smoothie." This enchanting concoction captures the essence of blooming hibiscus flowers, marrying their delicate flavour with a medley of fruits for a sip that's both refreshing and floral. Immerse yourself in the floral symphony and let each sip transport you to a garden in full bloom.

**Ingredients:**

**Hibiscus Tea (one cup, chilled):** Infuses the smoothie with the captivating floral notes of hibiscus.

**Strawberries (1/2 cup, hulled):** Add a burst of sweetness and a hint of tartness.

**Peach (one, peeled and sliced):** Enhances the floral profile with a juicy and fragrant peach.

**Orange (one, peeled and segmented):** Introduces citrusy brightness to complement the floral tones.

**Chia Seeds (one tablespoon):** Provide a nutrient boost and add a delightful texture.

**Method of Preparation:**

**Hibiscus Elixir:** Brew hibiscus tea and let it chill for a refreshing floral base.

**Strawberry Symphony:** Blend hulled strawberries to create a luscious berry puree.

**Peachy Harmony:** Add sliced peach to the mix, blending for a velvety consistency.

**Citrus Dance:** Incorporate peeled and segmented orange, which infuses a burst of citrusy notes.

**Chia Infusion:** Sprinkle chia seeds into the blend, stirring gently for a delightful texture.

**Benefits:**

**Floral Delight:** Experience the enchanting taste of blooming hibiscus flowers.

**Vitamin Rich:** Strawberries, peaches, and oranges contribute vitamins for a nourishing sip.

**Textural Sensation:** Chia seeds add a delightful crunch, enhancing the overall drinking experience.

Savour the Blooming Hibiscus Bliss Smoothie, a floral symphony in every sip that invites you to bask in the beauty of nature's blossoms.

# Concluding Note

As we reach the final pages of "Irresistible Detox Elixirs," I extend my heartfelt gratitude for joining me on this flavoursome expedition toward better health. Throughout this book, we've journeyed through a vibrant array of detox drinks, each sip contributing to the cleansing of our bodies and the enrichment of our overall well-being.

In this compilation, we've explored the refreshing depths of Phyto Smoothie Green Detox Juice, the invigorating and stimulating properties of Immune Booster Detox, and the delightful blend of flavours in the Cilantro Fiesta Drink. From the tangy notes of Berry Ginger Detox to the earthy warmth of Detox Haldi Tea, every recipe has been crafted with the dual purpose of detoxification and pleasure.

As you've immersed yourself in these recipes, I hope you've discovered new and delicious ways to nurture your body and gained insights into the science behind detoxification. The journey has been as much about education as it has been about indulgence.

Remember, the power to transform your health lies in your hands, or rather, in your glass. These drinks are not just beverages; they are self-care rituals and expressions of love for your body and well-being. Incorporating them into your routine can be a small yet significant step toward a healthier, more vibrant life.

I encourage you to experiment with these recipes, tailor them to your taste, and make them a delightful part of your daily routine. Whether you find solace in the comforting warmth of Honey Lemon Ginger Tea or the zesty kick of Ginger Explosion Detox, let these drinks be a source of joy in your wellness journey.

Thank you for entrusting me with a role in your pursuit of health and happiness. May every sip remind you of the beautiful balance between nourishment and enjoyment. Here's to your well-being, the love you have poured into yourself, and the delicious path ahead. Cheers to a healthier, happier you!

Thank you

# Other books by the Author

1. **Vitamins & Minerals:**

Unlock vibrant health with the essential guide to vitamins and minerals! Explore their benefits, rich food sources, daily recommendations, and expert insights on managing deficiencies and avoiding excesses.

2. **Arthritis is Reversible**

Shatter the Myths, Embrace Hope: Your Guide to a Brighter Future with Reversible Arthritis

Unmask the misconceptions and discover natural solutions for managing and potentially reversing arthritis.

3. **Detox Your Body (free E-book, available on author's website)**

Unveil your body's natural potential! detox to eliminate toxins, discover the signs and benefits and explore a range of safe and effective methods for lasting transformation.

Embrace a vibrant you. Learn why detox matters, identify the need, unlock amazing benefits, and delve into practical strategies for internal cleansing and revitalization.

**Forthcoming Titles**

- Knocking Depression with Food
- Healing Wonders: Nature's Miracles Unveiled
- Decoding Diabetes-Exploring the Real Cause
- Decoding Diabetes-The Path To Reversal
- Optimizing the Body's Repair Time: Harnessing the Power of Healing
- Fuel Your Life: The Ultimate Guide to Optimal Health and Vitality.

www.ingramcontent.com/pod-product-compliance
Ingram Content Group UK Ltd.
Pitfield, Milton Keynes, MK11 3LW, UK
UKHW020050200726
13845UKWH00055B/629

9 789334 078909